REAL LIFE SUPERMAN

The Training Guide to Become
Faster, Stronger & More Jacked
than 99% of the Population!

Vol. 1: Strength & Conditioning

---

by Markus A. Kassel

Disclaimer: this book is meant for information and educational purposes only. Consult with your physician before attempting any of the exercises described in this book or before making any drastic changes to your diet. The author will not be held accountable for any damage caused by the implementation of the advice given throughout this guide. Though the author found success with this method, results may vary from person to person.

First Edition.

Visit the author's website: http://RealLifeSuperman.com

Table of Contents

Introduction: Superheroes and the Quest for Perfection

When I was a kid, I'd go to sleep every night, counting the days on my tiny fingers until the next Friday. Not that I wanted more time to play video games or that I wished to be through with school; I was just eager to meet back with one of my heroes.

Every week, I'd be glued to the television, waiting feverishly for my new episode of the Incredible Hulk. I'd grab a bowl of popcorn and stare at the screen – with eyes as big as my pounding heart – as the puny little Bruce would unleash the beast and turn into a muscular behemoth that knew no limits! I couldn't help but wonder: what if it could be me in his busted shoes?

In those days, the Internet hadn't yet gone global and video rental shops like Blockbuster were only an option if you had the financial means to buy a VCR. That meant I couldn't get my hands on other TV shows or movies to feed my superhero needs. So, ultimately, I turned to comics.

From Spiderman's adventures to the Fantastic 4 and Superman, I devoured those stories that brought excitement to a life that – although peaceful and happy – was way too monotonous for the big dreamer that I was. I immersed myself in those colorful pages, imagining it was me flying in the air, saving the day against all odds.

More than the reunion with the Green Angry Giant, the weekends would also mean a trip to the supermarket. While my mother would be gathering the groceries, I'd wait at the book section, trying to make up my mind on the Fighting Fantasy gamebook I'd be spending my allowance on. What would I choose to be for this week? A mighty warrior, a wise wizard, a ninja master?

Now that I think about it, I don't believe that the feats of power and courage displayed by these heroes could explain by themselves why I felt so strongly attracted to them. There was something else at play here. I envied their destiny, no matter how tragic; the way they lived their existence outside the boundaries regular folks subjected themselves to. I admired the intensity with which they spent every moment of every day, and their willingness to put it all on the line to save the innocent. Because, despite their powers, they remained mortals who could be slain...

Those extraordinary, purposeful destinies violently clashed with what I saw around me. When I took a look at grown-ups in the streets, all I could sense was boredom and bitterness. Seldom did I notice any spark to light their dark and miserable lives. It made me realize, quite early, that I didn't want to follow in their footsteps. I wanted a path larger than life; a superhero fate where I could be anything I wished to be.

When I reached puberty, that fascination turned into a desire for action. I came to the conclusion that if my eyes could never shoot lasers, if adamantium claws would never spring out of my bare hands, it didn't mean I had to settle for this dull existence or the imaginary worlds inside my head. I could still take the matter in my own hands and become the master of my destiny. By training my body and my mind, I could rise above the rest and come as close as possible to developing superpowers.

I took up martial arts, starting with karate, then I added kickboxing to the mix to improve my hitting power and mental toughness. I still remember, aged 15, the first time I entered the ring in a 3x2 minutes amateur bout. How scared I was, waiting in the locker room for my turn to get beat up. I had a million butterflies in the stomach, a furious need to run away and not look back... But I survived that fight, and it showed me that fear was but an illusion. A smokescreen.

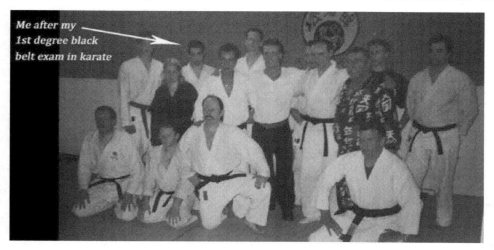

Me after my 1st degree black belt exam in karate

Working out 5 days a week now, I was investing all my pocket money in training books. That's how I discovered ancient practices like Qi Gong and Zen meditation that I incorporated into my program to try and get that extra edge. As my body hardened, I continued to challenge myself mentally. Meditation helped, but forcing myself to talk to girls was the hardest part for this tough-looking but shy at heart teenager.

As a young adult, I turned to body weight training to address my weaknesses and increase both my strength and body control. The same spirit would drive me, a couple years later, to engage in gymnastics and parkour. In the end, I would try everything that could potentially enhance my abilities and mental fortitude.

With all those training sessions, programming and fine-tuning, time flew by like a night out with your buddies, drinking beer and remaking the world. High school quickly became a memory and I had to think about my future. I went for a Masters in Communications, which I followed with a degree in Psychology. Even in my academic studies, it seemed like I was searching for answers. Maybe I thought that those classes would give me another, more scientific look into the inner workings of the human brain. Maybe I thought that, those diplomas in hand, I would unlock the secret to a super, invincible mind. To my huge dismay, I found out that they wouldn't.

Although I learned a lot of interesting facts, from the imprinting process discovered by Konrad Lorentz to the Invisible Gorilla experiment, those years of cramming didn't expand my horizons as I had hoped they would. And so continued my quest into adulthood...

One might imagine that this fixation would have faded by then. That this was just a temporary feeling, the fleeting fantasy of a kid in need of adrenalin. However, the older I got, the stronger I felt about it! Every fiber of my being was screaming for me to pack my bags and leave on some wild trip around the globe. I needed adventure. I needed to live like the superheroes of my childhood, with passion and intensity.

When you think about it, as kids, we possess that innate faculty to build incredible worlds and to inhabit them. It's second nature. But as we grow up, we end up losing more than our innocence; we become jaded, fearful animals that care way too much for the opinion of others.

Drawing from my foundations, I would up the ante and start living my own adventures through mud runs, street workouts, bushcraft and the likes.

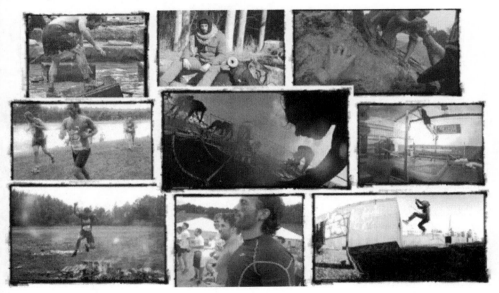

Now in my thirties, I've come a long way since those days I read comics under a blanket with a flashlight... but I know that the journey I'm on is never-ending. I keep pushing the envelope, putting myself in the direst situations not only to see how I'll react but also to increase my ability to adapt. I sleep in the wild, with a campfire for sole companion; I take part in CrossFit competitions; I run, jump, crawl, swim, laugh, learn, lose myself and rediscover my inner child... And while doing all this, I'm having a blast!

Now, you may be reading my story and begin to wonder whether I'm going to suggest you undergo the same tortuous process to reach your goals. If that's the case, let me put your mind at ease. Though this program is designed to make you superior on all levels, you won't have to suffer through the same ordeal. I already did it for you! Here, you won't have to experiment to

7

find what works and what doesn't. I'll give you nothing but actionable advice that'll make you more athletic, stronger and smarter by the week. I'll make your time and efforts count.

The goal of this series is to develop your full potential, to open your eyes to the world of possibilities that lies ahead, no matter your age or where you are at this particular moment in life. Whether it's a **superhero body** you want, the strength of a Juggernaut or the willpower of our favorite X-Men, this program will lead you there.

All I'm asking in return is for 100 days of your life. Commit to this program for 100 days and you'll become a new man! This is the promise I make to you.

What You'll Get with This Program: a Comprehensive Method

The title of this book wasn't chosen at random. If you've read through the intro, you know all about my fascination for superheroes and that burning desire to resemble them in every way possible. You also know how I've come to develop my training methods and why I strongly believe that I can get you in better shape than 99% of the population.

I realize that this might sound like a bold statement but, when you think about it, it's not such a far-fetched idea. The truth of the matter is that most people are in bad shape. Just sit down on a bench and observe men and women passing by. How do they look? How do they move? You don't have to go to the beach to witness the ravages of obesity. Even through their thick clothes, hunchback and shuffling gait, you can see how unhealthy average people have become.

But what about those who work out? you ask. Well, unfortunately, they seldom know squat about training and how the human body really works. They either follow the same, useless routine month after month and get confused as to why they're not making any progress. Or they try to copy bodybuilding pro's and jump from one program to the other, believing that their latest issue of "Muscle & Fitness" holds the key to a Greek god body.

All in all, out of every 100 people, 99 either do not train or follow a suboptimal plan that translates into less than stellar results.

One huge problem with most programs is that they're just plain BO-RING. Get on the elliptical and pedal away until you fall asleep, or go from machine to machine trying not to commit suicide as concentration curls lead to leg extensions and lateral raises. No wonder that a great deal ends up quitting after a while!

The best way to ensure that you not only stick to your training but that it delivers on the results is to make it fun, short and challenging. This is how I train and how I built my physique. This is the superman road to success that I'll share with you in this book.

By following my principles, you'll become faster, stronger and more jacked than everyone else around you. You'll have gained such athleticism that, in comparison to them, it'll seem like **you do have real superpowers**!

Now if the ultimate goal of this series is to elevate your game on all fronts – from learning to clear obstacles to withstanding pain and fighting –, we couldn't possibly cover it all in one book. We have to set our priorities straight. In the same manner that we can't be expected to run before we walk, we first have to prepare our body for what will come next.

The aim of this first installment will thus be to develop a fit body through conditioning, which will allow you to acquire other physical skills more rapidly afterwards. Learning to throw punches won't do you any good if you can't jump up and down for 3 seconds without having to stop to catch your breath! You need to increase your strength, your resilience and stamina.

This particular book will be divided in 5 sections that each deals with a critical component of your metamorphosis.

- **Part I – The Right Way to Eat for Performance**: in this chapter, we'll say a few words on nutrition and why you can't neglect that side of the equation if you're to make any sensible progress;
- **Part II – Turn into a Cardio Beast**: here, we'll detail the different exercises to consider in order to shed the fat and become a lean & mean machine;
- **Part III – Build Muscle with Strength Training**: adding muscle mass while increasing our overall strength will be the point of focus in this piece;
- **Part IV – Putting It All Together**: this is where we'll lay out our foolproof "100 days to a Super you" program, step by step;
- **Part V – Fine Tuning**: all the extra questions pertaining to recovery, sleep, motivation and so on will find an answer in this part.

I don't know about you but I for one cannot wait to get started! Talking about all this has just finished whetting my appetite. So, without further ado, let's discover how to get you the super physique you deserve!

PART I

The Right Way To Eat for Performance

"Eating is primal, Kara. That's why people make such a big deal out of where they sit, who with, and what they eat. It defines you, in a lizard brain way."

Owen Mercer (Captain Boomerang)

Wolverine may get away with drinking beers by the keg and smoking cigars like they're part of his therapy but he possesses amazing healing powers. You DON'T.

If your plan is to get in the best shape of your life, you need to lead a healthy and active lifestyle, and it all starts with bringing your nutrition under control.

The Optimal Diet

In a perfect world, what you eat would not only help you lose fat, it would promote muscle synthesis and increase your performance. When you go grocery shopping, you don't necessarily think about the impact every food item you put into your cart will have on your abilities. You don't start linking that chocolate bar to an increased likelihood of diabetes or that bottle of soda to sluggishness and lower levels of testosterone. Yet, every choice you make will either serve to liberate or limit you in the end.

Some experts go as far as stating that nutrition accounts for 70% of your results, while the remaining 30% depend on your exercising. I might not agree 100% with those numbers (a 50/50 split would be more accurate in my opinion) but the point is that your feeding habits remain highly critical. Not only because what you eat influences your body composition but also because it often dictates how you feel and behave. As the saying goes, we are what we eat, ain't we?

A great deal of the population maintains an unhealthy relationship with food. A relationship of dependency. At the store, we go from aisle to aisle, imagining how great that ice cream will taste when we'll dig into it and that its soft caramel core melts on our tongue. We imagine the satisfaction we'll experience from sinking our teeth into that juicy hamburger. The main motivation that drives us is pleasure, period. We have become complete slaves to these feel-good products, and that's the chief problem with our society. To add insult to injury, most diets completely overlook that factor of causality.

When you strive to lose weight, the typical scenario has you restrain yourself from the moment you open your eyes. You return to bed entirely famished and try not to think about the constant hunger that's gnawing at your guts. You try to put on a brave face but those foods haunt you like the ghost of a deceased relative. You see them dancing behind your closed eyelids, teasing you, tormenting you. It's a recipe for disaster.

Even with the best will in the world, you're bound to fail. No one can resist temptation forever. The key to continued success is to change the way you approach the whole thing. You need to start seeing the implications and ramifications of your every meal choice. You need to start viewing food as an ally, not an enemy that ought to be fought. But how is one supposed to achieve that goal, you ask?

Well, for one, we're under the assumption that the problem is psychological, that the cravings we suffer originate from inside our heads. This is a very dangerous belief as it puts the entire responsibility on your willpower. And when you give in and start binging, which will eventually happen, you think you have no one else to blame but yourself. You feel guilt creep in, watching that empty bag of chips lying on the kitchen table. "Why am I so weak? Why can't I resist?" you admonish yourself. The truth is that it might not be entirely your fault. Something may have forced your hand!

The truth is that **there's also a physical component to the dependency**. But before we address that issue and see how to manipulate our feeding to get rid of those urges (and feel better than we ever have before), we need to learn a little more about the way our body functions. The more we'll know about digestion, nutriments and their corollaries, the better equipped we'll be to make them work FOR us, instead of against!

The Science of Fat Loss

If you ever went to a Weight Watchers' reunion or read through a women's magazine, you might think that you've already uncovered the secret to a dream figure. As they all claim, you simply have to eat less calories than you burn to lose weight and regain your health, right? Not so fast, Maximoff!

While that's what I've been led to believe for a very long time, I found out after much searching that the picture wasn't completely accurate. Stories abound of people trimming down, eating nothing but pizzas or McDonald's, which may help support the "a calorie is a calorie" thesis... But there's always a trade-off to losing fat in such a manner. Whether it's the increase in triglycerides, the bad acne or the pounding headaches, there's always a price to pay. Somehow, it's like changing a flat tire on your car and breaking the radiator while doing so.

If your goal is to thin down, ward off sickness and perform like a champ, not all foods and calories are created equal. You see, digestion is not a simple process where everything you eat undergoes the same treatment. Some foods will be absorbed quickly; others will take more time. Some foods will cause the release of hormones; others won't. And when you learn that certain of those hormones may tinker with your hunger and feeling of satiety, you realize that putting the wrong ingredients on your plate may seriously harm your chances of success. That it may trick our bodies into believing we still need more food!

If you end up ingesting more calories than you consume, it's true that you'll gain weight. But this statement isn't 100% valid because it takes too pragmatic an approach to the matter. It reduces it to a simple numbers game, as if we were cold, calculating machines that could just follow our required quota without fail.

It totally omits the most important question that is: **why do we overeat in the first place?** Why can't we just eat our meal and be content with it? Once again, we go back to the question of addiction and dependency. To better understand how these two constantly plot to ruin our best efforts, let's see how energy enters the body at the molecular level and the different reactions it can generate depending on the macronutrients present.

Carbs

Carbs (short for carbohydrates) represent the first type of energy. They include sugars and starch, from those found in bread and pasta to those contained in fruits and rice. I won't bore you with their chemical properties as they bear little impact on the subject at hand but it's interesting to note that they're usually categorized as either simple sugars – called monosaccharides – or complex compounds known as polysaccharides.

Carbs reign supreme in the Western world. If the recommended intake ranges from 45% to 65% of our daily calories, the actual percentage may be much higher for most people. Just think about a typical day of eating for the average Joe... He wakes up, wolfs down a bowl of Lucky Charms with a glass of orange juice. At lunch, it's a chicken salad sandwich with a bag of chips, and a can of soda to wash it all down. And to close the day in perfect fashion, if Joe doesn't hit the closest fast-food joint when he gets off work, he'll cook a quick pot of pasta and be done with it (and let's not even get started on what he'll eat in front of the tube!)

As you can tell, carbs are everywhere and inseparable from our modern way of life. They're always cited as the primary form of energy for us, humans. And understandably so, seeing they represent the principal source for creating glycogen – a muscle and liver stored polysaccharide which serves as the preferred fuel of the brain and the muscles under intense effort.

But the main point of interest with sugars is the hormonal response they induce. When you eat carbs, the sugars get broken down in the stomach and pass into your bloodstream. The problem is that high blood glucose (hyperglycemia) is toxic. It interferes with the normal functioning of proteins in the blood and clog arteries, which can lead to cardiovascular diseases.

So, as a reaction, the pancreas produces insulin to chase the harmful molecules away and get the glucose levels back to normal (that's how glycogen is made, by the way.) But the production of insulin may eventually put a strain on the liver if loads of sugar keep coming and coming. In this case, the liver might start failing on its other duties. Fatty liver disease may ensue, with insulin resistance and other such nasty complications we could really do without.

As you're slowly starting to uncover, eating carbs in large proportions (as prescribed by most nutritionists) may be part of the problem. Which prompts the following question: if it gets in the way of optimum health, does it really have its place in a Superman's diet?

Proteins

Proteins, on the other hand, serve as the building blocks for our body. When repairs have to be done or new tissues ought to be fabricated, the organism turns itself to proteins. If you're looking to pack on muscle, they'll be your best ally. Like Mjolnir to Thor.

Where carbs get broken down into simple sugars during digestion, proteins will give off amino acids. It's those AAs that will be reassembled later on to create one of thousands potential proteins, depending on the particular needs of the body at that time. They can be used to fuel the body as well, when you get low on carbs and fats.

Of the myriad AAs available, only 9 can't be produced by the human body. You have to get them from the outside world, that is through eating, and that's why they're called "essential." Any type of meat should provide the whole 9 acids in sufficient amounts, so it usually poses no problem (unless you're a vegetarian, in which case you'll have to combine various legumes to ensure you show no deficiencies.)

On the hormonal side, proteins do not cause the release of problematic substances such as insulin. In fact, it'd be quite the opposite. When you consume proteins, the only notable hormone to make its way to your bloodstream is peptide YY which slows down your digestion and reduces your appetite. A very welcome hand if you're looking to lose weight!

Last but not least, proteins promote anabolism which – despite its fancy name – is nothing else than the synthesis of new proteins (or muscle tissue, as far as we're concerned.)

Fats
Of all the macronutrients, fats have to be the ones that get the worst rap. They're accused of causing all sorts of diseases and of being at the root of the obesity epidemic that's affecting our regions.

The truth of the matter is that they constitute an essential part of a healthy diet. Not only are they needed to assimilate soluble vitamins such as vitamin A, D, E, K and K2, as well as proteins; they also increase bone density, better our immune system, and – despite what most people believe – help better our cholesterol.

It's a widely held view that eating fat makes you fat, and that it puts you at risk of developing heart disease. However, when fat reaches the digestive track, it's not that thick, greasy product anymore that everyone imagines will spread and clog our arteries. Under the release of lipase and bile, fat will emulsify and result in fatty acids that will be transported through our blood, just like other molecules.

In the same vein, even though they contain 9 calories per gram (versus 4 for carbs and proteins), fats are remarkably filling. Overeating on fats alone can prove to be a real challenge, unlike what happens with sugar.

What we need to remember from this chapter is that to keep our body happy and retain control over our food consumption, we had better try and **limit insulin secretion**. This will be, as we'll see later down the road, one of the keys to building a lean and muscular physique.

Anabolism and the Road to Bigger Muscles
While we're on the subject of muscle building, as we hinted above, you'll need a diet that's rich in protein. There's a good reason Weider, Optimum and other supplements companies have made a fortune selling protein powder. It works. Pay attention to the buff guys at the gym, once they're done working out. 9 times out of 10, you'll see them reaching in their bag to pull out a shake.

Now, if proteins are needed for the body to create new tissue, it's almost impossible to maintain an anabolic state 24/7. In fact, the body is constantly switching between building and destroying, anabolism and catabolism… The only way to have the anabolic state linger on is to either pump yourself full of steroids (in which case, you can stop reading this book right away because you don't care about your health and developing your true potential) or to go in bodybuilder's mode and eat every 2-3 hours (which means waking up at 3 a.m. to chew on some chicken breast or down a vanilla shake.) But even that last option is not without obvious downsides.

The bottom line is that, unless you plan on competing in Mr. Olympia and become as slow and stiff as a bird caught in an oil spill, neither is necessary. If what you're after is an athletic build; a toned body that feels as great as it looks and which shows great functionality, there's only one moment where anabolism truly matters: right after training.

Following your strength session, your body will go into high gear to repair the "damage" you've caused. It'll boost testosterone production to fix the micro-tears that will have appeared over your muscle fibers. This will open a window of opportunity during which protein synthesis will be highly facilitated. Make it count!

If there ever was a moment to eat carbs, this would be it. Ingesting sugars with your protein will maximize your results as the insulin spike helps push those sweet amino acids into your legs and pecs to make them grow.

This highlights the importance of including protein-rich foods in our diet. Foods like fish, poultry, beef, game and eggs. But it also highlights the necessity of steering clear of products known to increase estrogen levels (a female sex hormone which impedes the natural production of testosterone.)

For a detailed plan of what to eat and what to stay away from, refer to Part IV of this book.

Fuel for Performance

So far we've learned that, to lean down and add some meat to our frame, we'll have to regulate our insulin secretion and learn to love our protein. But what about performance? What should we add to the groceries list to have our body operate at its best?

In a way, food is like the fuel you pump into a car. Go for cheap, low quality gas and not only will you be unable to push it to the extreme, you'll greatly reduce its longevity. You put garbage in, you get garbage out. It's the same with food.

The first priority should be to guarantee sufficient intake of fruits and vegetables. Your mom was right all along; you need to eat your veggies to become a big and strong boy! The slightest deficiency in vitamins, minerals or other micronutrients can affect your recovery and your sleep, cause you pain in the joints, weaken your bones, induce a depressive state or even damage your nerves! By neglecting your greens, you'd also miss on precious antioxidants that help fight off infections, illnesses, and cancer among other things.

Secondly, you had better skimp on the goodies that lead to apathy, fatigue and weakness. When food is hard to assimilate and/or full of toxins – as is the case with junk food – your body will divert much of its energy to dealing with digestion. Which leaves little for you to break any record!

Our food choices should ultimately allow us to go hard and to keep going when most other organisms would've quit. There's no denying that your mental will play a huge part in helping you push past your limits but, without proper nutrition to begin with, you won't even get to the point where the mind should take over. You'll have long crumbled to pieces. Which brings us to an important matter: if carbs need to be kept in check as far as insulin is concerned, how to make sure our performance won't suffer? Where will we be getting our energy from?

Those are some of the questions that left me scratching my head as I was searching for the perfect diet. I had to find the subtle balance that would allow me to meet every one of my criteria. Here's how I came to develop my eating habits. Here's my food story.

You Can Have Your Cake and Eat It Too (well, almost)

Fingers Burnt & Lessons Learned

When it comes to nutrition, much like training, I've tried it all from one extreme to the other. I would read about a new technique and get all fired up, thinking I had finally found the key to unlock my full potential... but, one after the other, each method quickly showed its shortcomings.

When I experimented with several days of fasting, although it brought clarity of mind and an improved ability to focus, it made me weak and lose muscle mass. The same occurred with calorie restriction. No energy left.

Eating like a bodybuilder, that is every 2-3 hours, didn't prove to be much better. It made me bloated like heck and never truly satisfied. I did put on some muscle under that diet but it didn't help one bit with fat reduction. And let's not even talk about the gas, the ever-present gas! I was looking to become a superhero, but not Fartman! Boy was it uncomfortable! To sum up, it didn't make me feel good at all.

On a side note, if you're into bodybuilding, that's great as it'll give you a nice head start. However, with this book, I'm looking to offer you more than a great physique. Whereas bodybuilding is all about getting as muscular as possible (often without any regard for health), here we're not only aiming for a body that will make heads turn but that will continue to do so until you die of old age! We're not planning to end up like most pro BB'ers who spend their last decades paying for all the abuse they put their body through.

Anyways, back to the subject at hand. If today, I've finally managed to strike the ideal compromise, you can notice from my story that it hasn't been easy. It was, in fact, a very long road. You see, I grew up like most kids, loving my sweets and hating those awful veggies. Every Saturday, my brother and I would put the squeeze on our mother to go and have our burger and fries at our favorite spot. She'd cut my burger in two, and I'd eat each half in complete silence as if in communion with God. I also remember those evenings when we'd eat dinner with nothing but a bag of chips in front of a good movie. Or those trips to the local market where we'd buy candy by the pound.

I won't lie, more than 20 years later, they're still among my most vivid and powerful memories. I can still smell the fried onions, the taste of barbecue sauce on my tongue... As if that food had left an indelible mark deep inside my core.

That sweet tooth and attraction for fatty foods didn't become a problem until I was twelve years old. As you know from the introduction, I was a very active kid. That extra energy I absorbed never found its way to my waistline because I was burning it all, running, jumping and having fun. But soon after my 12th birthday, I had a car accident. With a double leg fracture, brain concussion and busted arm, I was sidelined for nearly 6 months. It would've been but a dent in my journey if I hadn't continued to feed like a lumberjack after a day out in the woods. That year, I put on serious weight... and it sure as hell wasn't muscle!

When I resumed sports, I had that much more motivation. To resemble my heroes, not only did I need to become stronger and more resistant, I now also had to get rid of that disgracious padding that had taken residence in my belly. It would take me years to evict the unwelcome squatter.

In my personal library, next to my comics, martial arts guides, training manuals and Fighting Fantasy issues, I was now collecting every nutrition book I could put my hands on. Thanks to those, I learned how the body works, the role of vitamins and macronutrients, the importance of sufficient hydration... Relying on those readings, I tested what made sense, discarded conflicting info. And the years passed. Eventually, by trial and error, and fine-tuning my food logs, I found some kind of balance that allowed me to stay relatively fit... but not yet 100% healthy.

Time for a little confession: I've always been kind of an extremist in everything I do. Whether it be working on a project, playing videogames, learning a new craft or a new sport, eating, you name it; when I like something, I'll often overindulge. And it was the same with my lifelong love affair with sweets. For the entire week, I'd eat super strict then, come Saturday, I'd let loose like a starved pig in a free buffet. I'd eat chips, chocolate, cookies, ice cream, pastries... and the main culprit: candy.

It made me feel like crap, both physically (due to the massive insulin dump) and mentally, but I kept doing it, week after week, year after year, stuck in an abusive relationship. Come to think about it, it wasn't love that made me fall every time. It was addiction. I needed my shoot of pure, unadulterated sugar and I couldn't picture my life without it.

The superhero wannabe had become a total slave to his passions. As with the accident, this could've been but a regrettable setback if I had made good progress during the rest of the week. Unfortunately, I wasn't. Although I followed every rule in the book – calculating my macros to get the right amounts of fats, carbs and proteins –, although I ate good portions, I felt famished and tired all the time. I'd check my watch every five minutes to see how long I still had to wait until the next plate of chicken with rice. My training wasn't going anywhere either. I had hit a plateau that I couldn't seem to get through no matter what I tried.

I knew something had to be done eventually, but what? Nothing worked. The deliverance would, once again, come from my readings. One day, flipping through a scientific journal, I stumbled upon an article retracing the changes in our diet through time, from the dawn of mankind to the 21st century. I read how, for millions of years, we had lived as hunters-gatherers; how our bodies had evolved to thrive in that environment. And how we had switched to our modern carb-heavy diet only a few millennia ago, with a huge rise in cancer, cardiovascular disease and diabetes. Illnesses our ancestors were completely free of.

As I kept furthering my research, I found out that adopting the ways of hunters-gatherers could bring more than protection against present-day ailments. I found out that some people actually followed those precepts today and that they were seeing dramatic improvements in their health, body composition and ability to perform. That diet had a name: the paleo or caveman diet.

The Caveman Diet: Rediscovering Our Origins

The reasoning behind "eating paleo" goes something like this: when you take a timeline from the moment our species arose (around 2,000,000 years ago) and today, you can see that we've only been feeding on agricultural products such as corn and wheat for less than 0.5% of our existence.

If you're up-to-date with the evolution theory, you know that it takes a lot of time and mutations for organisms to adapt and change. In those tiny 10,000 years that separate our era from that of the agricultural revolution – which marked the real shift towards our current diet –, our bodies didn't have the opportunity to learn how to deal with those new foods. We are, thus, not (yet?) physiologically suited for this grain-based diet we've been trying to force on ourselves, as is apparent from the different health troubles we must deal with on a daily basis. We've become pale images of our strong, vibrant and energetic forebears.

By reverting back to our pre-agricultural ways, the proponents of the caveman diet hope to reclaim that lost heritage. They're aiming to eat nothing but foods our body evolved to thrive on. Basically: meat, fish, vegetables, nuts, fruits, berries and the occasional tuber. Now, one might argue that those products varied greatly depending on the location we found ourselves in – a forest providing a different selection than say a savannah or a patch of land near the coast. But the broad lines remained identical: meat and wild plants.

And no carbs (except for those present in fruits, veggies and the odd sweet potato.)

Knowing that, could it be that the decline in our health during these last millennia stemmed from the addition of sugar?

The Case against Sugar

As suggested by the paleo concept, our bodies might not be made for subsisting on huge loads of carbs like they actually do. We've already described what happens to us every time we eat sugars; the pancreas releases insulin to push the glucose out of the bloodstream and store it as glycogen inside the liver or the muscles. But what if the stocks are already full? What if, because you rely too much on your oats and noodles, you can never use up your glycogen bank and still you keep the deliveries coming in like pumpkin trucks to the supermarket on Halloween's eve? The answer is simple.

Little by little, your muscle cells will develop a resistance to the insulin. They'll block the passage and prevent any entry. Still having to deal with this glucose in excess, the pancreas will work twice as hard, secreting even more insulin. At this stage, out of options, the insulin will have no other choice but to lead the glucose to the only other type of cells available: your beloved fat. That's how you'll build layer upon layer of lard. Not because you've binged on bacon and butter but because you wouldn't slow down with the cereals and the sugary yoghurt!

It bears repeating: when you get spanked by your general practitioner because your triglycerides have reached new heights, it's the sugar that's to blame. Not the fat!

You might be frowning at this point. What I'm telling you probably goes against everything you've been told. What about the glycemic index? Aren't complex carbs supposed to be assimilated differently than simple sugars? Aren't they supposed to produce a much lesser insulin reaction and, therefore, be less harmful?

I see where you're coming from. I know, as that's what I've been led to believe and apply for years. However, in the end, after your digestive enzymes have accomplished their task, all carbs end up as glucose molecules... Molecules which need a way out, somehow.

The other main problem with carb-rich foodstuffs is that they're either highly processed (read devoid of much nutritional interest) or part of the grains family. Why is that an issue, you ask? Well, it all starts with gluten.

What is gluten and why it's bad for us: from animals to plants, the "adapt-or-die" pressure of evolution has always favored the survival of organisms that could protect themselves against their predators. Animals evolved to grow teeth, nails, claws, beaks, bones, as well as venom and poison.... and so did plants, in their manner. The difference is that plants couldn't take any physical action to defend themselves. So, they had to design other, more passive mechanisms that would preserve their integrity. Mechanisms such as spines and toxins. For grains, this resulted in the appearance of lectins and phytates... and the worst of them all: gluten.

If some animal species have in turn developed the ability to digest those harmful compounds without any side-effect, the same cannot be said about Man. Although you're probably not Celiac (in which case, you WOULD know of your intolerance to gluten), you may very well be part of the third of the population which is still very sensitive to its effects. In fact, nobody can eat it and say to show no adverse reaction. We're all concerned. For one, when gluten enters our digestive system, a serious inflammation ensues. The body treats it as a threat that ought to be squashed ASAP. To this end, it releases a stream of antibodies. Not cool! Where it gets even worse is that the gluten section responsible for the immune response looks a lot like other proteins synthetized by our vital organs. No need to spell out what's coming next. You guessed it: the antibodies will start unleashing their fury on the said organs! And that's how you damage your pancreas and develop type-1 diabetes. Isn't it lovely?

While they're at it, trying to stop the invasion, the antibodies will also attack your intestines. Little by little, they'll erode their walls, making them lose their waterproofness and leak bacteria and other such hazards inside your bloodstream!

As you can see, if insulin wasn't reason enough to limit your grains intake, gluten should definitely be. Grains wreak just too much havoc inside our guts. They literally put our health in danger.

Once again, I can see you raise an eyebrow. If grains are so bad, then how come the government doesn't inform the population? How come the majority of scientists advise to follow the regular food pyramid where carbs sit at the place of honor?

I don't want to sound like a conspiracy theorist (I prefer to leave government bashing to Magneto) but never lose sight of this reality: profit – and not the well-being of the population – will always remain the first priority for companies and corporations. And when you have two of the most powerful lobbies on the planet – namely pharmaceutics and agriculture – pressing you to push their agendas and good interests, you comply. Whoever you are. Even if you're the Head of State.

Maybe it's up to us, supermen in the making, to change the situation. One body at a time.

Why Paleo Meets My Criteria

When I first learned about all this, the returning to our prehistoric ways, the going against everything I had learned about nutrition in the last decade, I must admit I was kind of skeptical.

If I was feeling hungry right after my plate of meat with rice or pasta, wouldn't it get even worse if I replaced the carbohydrates with freaking broccolis? Those veggies wouldn't make me feel full but miserable; I would become drained and faded, like I did when I fasted non-stop for several days in a row, wouldn't I?

Another concern that was going through my mind pertained to deficiencies. Without this important macronutrient, wouldn't I sustain fiber, mineral or energy deficits? Although I knew the theory – that the foods I'd substitute for the carbs should meet all my needs –, it still seemed a little hard to swallow. I needed to see it with my own eyes, whether the paleo diet was all it claimed to be. As I had learned from experience: don't believe everything you read. Always put it to the test.

As I'd soon find out, my worries were groundless. After a few days of adaptation, paleo stabilized my hunger and filled me with a steady flow of energy. When you eat the regular Western diet with carbs as primary fuel, you're teaching your body to use sugars to function. Which is far from ideal as you're making it dependent on a resource that needs constant supplying. And when you can't deliver, well you suffer. You can't utilize all that fat you're carrying around as your body goes into some kind of tunnel vision and completely disregards your adipose tissue. As if you had a full tank of oil to heat up your house but no way to connect it to your home. Drowsiness and hunger ensue.

On the other hand, once you reduce your carbs and force your body to rely on fats, you don't have to worry about seesawing levels of efficiency anymore. You get your energy right from within, like it was meant to be!

Speaking from my own experience, shifting from carb to fat-burning translated into:

- An even lower body fat %. Even though I was already quite fit to begin with, I still managed to lose some lard while eating my fill and not having to make any additional efforts;

- More muscle mass, as all the meat I ate promoted anabolism and created the perfect environment for muscle growth;

- The total disappearance of those uncomfortable gases. No more having to endure painful tightness in the stomach. Just gone!

- A better looking skin, clearer and blemish-free;

- An improved quality of sleep and general well-being;

- More gustatory pleasure as I discovered the many joys of cooking (spices, stir-fried veggies...);

- Peace of mind as I didn't have to worry about counting calories or weighing my food anymore; I knew that everything that went through my mouth contributed somehow to making me a more efficient and healthy human being.

That's just some of the benefits I got out from the switch. Living paleo, though, isn't all about nutrition which is only the tip of the iceberg. Paleo is a way of life, an aspiration to live with as little stress and as much playtime as possible. We're not suggesting to adopt an "I don't give a %ù!*" attitude or to go all out hippie. It's a quest to find joy and happiness in everything you do. To take the time to enjoy the simple pleasures in our existence. That's a philosophy that deeply resonates with me.

With the dust settled, I can say that going paleo cured me of my addiction to sweets. I still indulge from time to time but it's become a deliberate choice (a piece of cake at a birthday party, a slice of pizza when out with a friend). I don't HAVE to have it like I did in the past. This is what I had been searching for all along. Real freedom of choice. Finally, I've become the master of my destiny!

How YOU Can Implement It Today
If I asked you right now to open your kitchen cabinet and to throw away anything vaguely connected to sugar, you'd probably tell me to go to hell, thinking you couldn't possibly survive without your loaf of bread or your oats.

But that would be the addict in you speaking. That would be the very voice which prevented you from accomplishing your dreams thus far.

It's about time we shut it up, put our money where our mouth is and reach for the top!

After about 10 days on this "diet", once you'll have weaned off carbs, you'll see that everything I'm telling you is right. The hunger will stop. The pounds will start to melt away. And you'll feel like Captain America just out of his transformation machine! An entirely new man. You'll notice that there was no reason to be afraid, that not only it's delicious and easy to eat like our ancestors; it also feels right on a very profound level. If you have one regret, it'll be not to have started sooner!

To help you on the road to a superior body, here are a few tips you can put into practice right away. Why wait? Use the momentum you've gathered through this book to make significant changes, not next week, not the day after tomorrow... but today!

By now, I think you got the message: the most important modification to your nutrition should be the ditching of grains and the inclusion of proteins & fats in every one of your meals. As much as possible, you should aim to eat meat and vegetables, with fruits, nuts and tubers every now and then.

But how are you supposed to track your progress? Even though we never count calories with this "diet" (as it's hard to overeat on this type of food, unlike with carbs), you might want to keep a journal in the beginning to note down everything you eat. That will not only act as a reminder that everything you take in should respect the paleo guidelines but it'll also help to fine-tune your plan. If you're not losing weight, maybe you're eating too many almonds. If you're feeling weak past the 2-3 weeks mark, maybe you're not using enough oils and fats. With a journal, you can refer back and see where the problem may lie. In short, less guesswork involved.

Secondly, in a perfect world, every meat, fish and vegetable you'd buy would either be grass-fed, wild caught or organic. But I know from experience that unless you're ready to take a mortgage on your house, you won't be able to afford it. Those products are just too costly. So, although it's not the very best option, you can still reap great rewards and reach your goals with their "regular" counterparts. Just make sure not to eat the fat of grain-fed animals as that's where all the toxins they've accumulated will be stored. Cut it with a knife and replace it with some coconut or olive oil.

Which brings us to one of the main hurdles to eating paleo: money. It's funny how, if you want to eat crap that'll make you fatter than Wilson Fisk, you can get tons of it for a couple of bucks, but if you want a healthy alternative that'll make you lean and strong, you almost have to take out a loan!

Fortunately, with a little thinking, you can find a few creative ways to start on a budget:

- **Grow your own veggies**: if you live in New York or don't have a garden, no worries. You can still (re)grow vegetables in glass jars! To do that, simply save your kitchen scraps and plant them in some soil. It works for garlic, onions, sweet potatoes, celery, and cabbage among other tasty things;

- **Buy in bulk**: this one is a no-brainer but purchasing your meat in bulk and storing it in the freezer for later can seriously cut the costs. To get the best prices, check the ads in your mail to see where they have interesting discounts that week (2 pounds free for 2 pounds bought, and so on);
- **Trade your steak for some organs**: kidneys, livers and hearts are not only cheap, they're also chock full of nutrients and vitamins. They may seem gross if you've never tried them but they're actually delicious when cooked right;
- **Participate in a co-op**: the concept is dead easy; donate time for food. Most organic co-ops are often on the lookout for extra pairs of hands. Be those hands. Anyways, superheroes are all about helping out, aren't they? So, if you can get nice organic food for your assistance, you kill two birds with one stone;
- **Search for products about to expire**: when walking down the aisles at your supermarket, look for items near the expiration date. Usually, they'll get a -20%, -30% or even -50% discount;
- **Go for canned food**: no, although cheap, pet food isn't part of our diet! When I mention canned food, I'm referring to tuna and salmon. With this option, you'll be able to grab wild caught fish that's full of omega 3's at a fraction of its regular cost.

Dozens of techniques exist to keep the bills low but this short list should be more than enough to get you started on the right foot. Take one or two of those and put them to good use.

"That's all well and good", you say, "but what am I exactly to eat?" I know it can be puzzling at first; it's one big change I'm asking you to make. But by keeping it simple, you'll ensure you stick to it. For example, to give you a rough idea of what to expect, here's what I eat on a typical day:

Breakfast: eggs & bacon (5 whole eggs, 4 strips of bacon.)

Lunch: monster salad (huge mixed salad with 2 cans of tuna, olives, tomatoes, capers, avocado, olive oil, lemon juice, salt and pepper.)

Dinner: juicy steak with butter, eggplants, zucchinis and a sweet potato.

Snacks: some almonds and walnuts + two squares of 85% dark chocolate.

I also fast once a week (generally on Mondays) to boost my testosterone production and immune system, as well as detoxify my organism. What's important with this method is that it remains occasional and that you never go over the 24 hours mark. After that, it gets counterproductive.

I don't recommend that you engage in fasting at first, though. I'm merely making the introduction as it'll become a useful tool in the later stages of your transformation. As for the recipes you can follow, I invite you to join me in Part V where we'll detail the whole program.

Speaking of program, now that we've gotten our nutrition under control, it's time to turn to the second essential piece of it: cardio training! Take a deep breath, and let's see how to develop a body that would make Colossus himself proud!

PART II

Turn Into a Cardio Beast

"Life is locomotion, if you're not moving, you're not living."

The Flash

Don't we all wish we could become superhero carbon copies by the push of a button? Like choosing our powers and the size of our biceps as we would a station on the radio? "Nah, I don't like that one. Next!"

Unfortunately, it takes time and dedication to succeed in this endeavor. One does not just grow muscle and explosiveness overnight. But you know what? I'm damn happy it's like that and not the other way around! Otherwise, every Joe and his neighbor would look like the Man of Steel. And how can you be "super" if there are no more regular guys?

Cardio training will be essential in our quest for multiple reasons, mainly to:

- Burn energy and lose weight;
- Increase our metabolism;
- Improve our stamina and overall performance.

All of which will work closely together to create a synergetic effect in which each component will be reinforced by the other in a mighty circle of awesomeness. When you train as I'll show you below, you'll lose weight, which in turn will make you more efficient, which in turn will raise your metabolism and will allow you to train even harder... and the cycle will keep on strengthening, feeding on itself. Isn't it just beautiful?

You'll understand now why cardio training is such a key element of our program. It'll be critical in helping us become the very best version of ourselves we can be. Moreover, on a pure physiological note, it'll enhance our respiratory capacity and strongly lower our risks of developing cancer or heart disease. As it works towards the same goals, it's the perfect companion to eating paleo!

However, to reap all those nice benefits, one still has to go about it the right way. Which, as we'll uncover, is far from a foregone conclusion...

The Traditional Approach

To lean down and get those stubborn abs to show, we have to pay attention to our diet (see Part I) and training regimen. That much we already know. But if most people still find a way to mess up their efforts with their eating habits, it's nothing compared to how badly they exercise!

Because they don't know better, they just emulate other folks at the gym. They don't stop one second to put two and two together and wonder: if those people on the elliptical – who're doing what I'm about to do – look nothing like the models of athleticism I praise, do I really want to follow in their footsteps?

No, they just hop on the next stationary bike, plug their headphones into the built-in screen, put the timer on 1h, and start cycling casually while watching a rerun of Breaking Bad.

They couldn't do worse.

In reality, 90% of people either train for too long or not with enough ferocity. And that's why so few of them succeed. When you try to gather all the different techniques that exist for cardiovascular training, you end up with a list as long as Mr. Fantastic's arms... and many of those will cause more harm than good in the long run! So, how are you to sort through this clutter? To be of help, your training needs to be challenging. It must push you both physically and mentally, and force you to change.

But if I'm here, assuming the lecturing role, I must say it took some hard lessons for me to finally see the light. As you probably have, I've done my share of screwing up too...

Cardio Beast in the Making

Before I start with the self-flagellation and tell you of the million ways in which I erred, I want to stress out that I do feel for those who're stuck in their cardio rut. The truth is that they're not responsible for their mistake. They're but the victims of hype and hearsay, following the latest fashionable trends or the same ineffective techniques our grand-parents were already falling for decades ago. They don't have hundreds of hours to invest to discover what truly works, so they put their trust in self-proclaimed authorities (like gym trainers) who're often in no better shape than those they're trying to coach.

I don't want you to suffer the same fate. I want you to get educated so as to become an expert in your own right who'll know what's best for him and the exact reasons why he's doing a particular workout. In short, I want you to take control and become your own man.

To show you that I understand how difficult the road can be, did you know that I too once followed the herd blindly? I thought that, to lose that lard which I had gained after my accident and to increase my stamina for my martial arts bouts, the best way would be to take up running. If so many people were doing it, it had to work, hadn't it?

I began with a dozen minutes, a mix of walking and running. I kept checking my pulse to try and stay within the famous "fat-burning" zone. Slowly but surely, the mileage increased and the time spent running as well. After a few months, I was running nonstop for an entire hour. Then for two. I was eating mile upon mile and burning more than 1,000 calories a run. But even if the fat was slowly coming off, my body was reacting in disturbing ways. For one, naive that I was, I thought running would contribute to building my legs. After all, I was hitting them strong, making their life miserable with all those kilometers; so they were bound to grow, weren't they? It turned out to be the total opposite! My quads were getting smaller and smaller. I was actually losing muscle mass!

My body cannibalized this hard-earned tissue to feed my runs. Not only that but I was experiencing serious pain in my joints. After 7-8 miles, my kneecaps would feel as if they were about to burst. I also developed nasty headaches that wouldn't go away unless I went to bed. And don't get me started on the poor state of my feet, numb and torn to shreds.

"What am I doing wrong?" I continued to ask myself, time and time again. I was playing by the book, making sure I stayed sufficiently hydrated, respecting the suggested distances... I couldn't figure it out. One thing was certain though, it definitely wasn't a pleasant affair. To go out and accomplish my duty, I had to muster all my strength. But not in the good sense of the word. Not like those times when you amp yourself up to break a personal record. More like having a tattoo on the ribs and trying to bite the bullet until it's over.

In the end, I wasted countless hours that I'll never get back. Thank God, I realized that the fault was in the running long distances itself and I stopped before the damage got too severe that I couldn't have undone it.

Now that I think back, years later, I can't help but wonder how I didn't understand it sooner. It's always easier to get the answer right in retrospect, when you have the advantage of past experiences. Running hundreds of kilometers per month, what was I thinking? Was I really trying to become a bag-of-bones marathoner? We both know I was rather inspired by the physique of sprinters, powerful and explosive.

That should've raised a red flag. But then, sometimes the most obvious truths are those that continue to elude you the longest...

The Many Perils of Prolonged Cardio

Let me sum things up in case you'd still have doubts: doing cardio at moderate intensity for hours on end will NOT help you reach your goals of ultimate fitness. In fact, it'll most probably prevent you from doing so! Prolonged cardio is a recipe for disaster.

Don't just take my personal story as proof; there are dozens of ways in which it can hinder your progress. For example, while you're busting your butt off, eating piles of meat and pushing weights to reach a perfect anabolic state, long distance running will come and stab you in the back by bringing your testosterone production all the way down. Good luck with adding a single ounce of muscle to your frame now!

The main problem with this type of training is that it puts the body under a lot of tension. When that strain is temporary, the body can bounce back and come back stronger. However, when it drags on for hours, cortisol will be released in great quantity. What does that mean? It means that this hormone of stress will produce free radicals and inflammation that will induce a toxic environment for your other cells. And when the inflammation occurs at a faster rate than your body can tend to, the destruction part of the equation prevails over the healing. Irremediable damage ensues.

Unfortunately for us, that's just the beginning of the nightmare. Cortisol secretion is also known to depress your immunity system, favor your ability to store abdominal fat, and break your precious muscle down. In other words, it's one super villain we ought to combat with all our might!

To make things worse, long-distance running may cause a hypertrophy of the heart in the long term which will make it weaker. And we can seldom say we've gone overboard until something finally happens to it (heart attack, anyone?) With other muscles like the legs, you don't have that sort of issue. You can feel – both physically and in your gut – when you've pushed too far. Should you persist and still continue, you'd risk a tear at worst. That would be too bad but you'd live. With the heart, I'm not so sure! Prolonged cardio may even cause memory loss in some people!

If you want to avoid those deleterious effects and become a real life superman, you know now that you'll need to approach your cardio training in a different manner. The way sprinters do.

HIIT or the Key to Super Performance

For the cardio part of our program, we'll thus turn to HIIT or High-Intensity Interval Training. Sprints are one way to go about it but there are as many possibilities as there are physical activities in that HIIT's principles can be applied to almost any sport.

In essence, you'll substitute quick and fierce bursts of effort for the longer more moderate type. You'll perform an exercise or series of exercises for a given set of minutes and with an intensity close to your maximum. Then, you'll rest. And repeat this cycle until you reach the end of the allotted time (rarely more than 20 minutes.)

In other words, you'll alternate short spurts of extreme energy where you'll go all out with periods of lower intensity which will allow you to catch your breath just enough to go at it again.

With this training, you'll become faster and more explosive. Your aerobic as well as anaerobic abilities will skyrocket, but that's not even the best "side effects" on the list. By limiting the time spent working out, you'll limit the release of cortisol as well as the wear and tear on your joints. You'll also make your metabolism shoot through the roof, with an "afterburn effect" that'll continue to burn calories hours after you've taken your shower and slipped into your favorite pj's. And all those calories expended, they'll come right from your fat. Not your muscle mass! More than offering a protection for your muscles, in fact, HIIT will give them a nice boost as human growth hormone production will rise from your movements' intensity!

All in all, HIIT is the ideal companion to start developing our super powers. It'll be like Bruce Banner's gamma rays, Peter Parker's spider bite, Hal Jordan's power ring to us… You'll have to hang in there as it'll get tough at times, but the benefits you'll gain will be worth all the pain. I can guarantee you that.

How to Get Started

To start on the right foot, you first ought to calculate/test your maximum performance. A lot of people who get into HIIT make the mistake of setting equal durations for their resting and exercising periods. They don't allow sufficient recovery time and, thus, find themselves unable to perform the next turn at full speed. Round after round, they get more and more tired, and the intensity plummets. Soon, they're not getting much out of their session anymore. They're just too darn exhausted.

Testing your maximum output will ensure you know how many reps of a given exercise you can chain together or how fast you can run before you crumble. That way, you can remain just below that threshold and never risk "running dry" before you're done. In the same spirit, you'll be planning enough rest between each burst (usually, 2 to 3 times that of your max effort.)

Some Options to Consider

With sprints, the obvious choice when it comes to HIIT, you'll begin with a warm-up of a few minutes. Once your muscles and joints are ready to rock, you'll run for 1 min 30 at medium intensity, before going full blast and maintaining the pace until 30 seconds have elapsed. With 6 rounds of both (for a total of 12 minutes), you should have your hands more than full if you have no prior experience of this type of training.

As you can witness, sprints are easy to put into practice yet highly effective. Nonetheless, it's always nice to have a few other alternatives up your sleeve to keep things interesting and continue challenging your limits.

Here are some variations I use:

Hill runs: you start yawning whenever you think about regular sprints? Been there, done that? If you want to take it up another notch, you can bring your runs to a hill. You'll discover a whole new world of possibilities. And hurting. On top of draining the oxygen out of your body like a dive into icy water, hill runs will give your calves and thighs one serious workout. Choosing the right hill is paramount. You want a slope that's just steep enough and neither too short nor too long.

To apply the HIIT principles to this exercise, go up the hill as fast as possible. Time your ascent to know how long it takes. Rest for 2-3 times that number. Then, do it again for a total of 6 rounds.

Rope jumping: this is one killer skill you should definitely pick up. Rope skipping will make you ultra-light on your feet and fast as lightning (think Muhammad Ali quick). It'll also improve your coordination and reflexes.

For your HIIT sessions, regular jumps won't do. They're just not demanding enough. To feel the burn, you'll have to up the pace by either performing double unders – if you can – or by raising the knees as high as you can. With rope jumping, I've found that you can't go as fast as with sprints, so you have to increase the time spent at full speed and decrease the resting in order to stay within our limits. Rounds that last 1 minute (20 seconds all out – 40 seconds at a slow pace) work great.

Rowing: if you have access to a rower, I strongly suggest adding some rowing to your program. Unlike running, it'll work your whole body. More muscle groups involved means more oxygen consumption, means more calories used and a deeper burn. This will have you beg for mercy.

One fun routine I like to go through is to row hard for 100m, rest 20 seconds; row hard for 200m, rest 40 seconds; row hard for 300m, rest 1 minute. Then, to do it again in reverse order: 300m – 1 minute; 200m – 40 seconds; 100m – 20 seconds.

Boxing: I don't often box for HIIT purposes because it's the least intense option of the bunch. Still, it makes for a welcome addition to your training when inserted between 2 hill run sessions for example. It'll be especially useful to train your hitting speed after you've learned the techniques I'll share with you in book II of this series dedicated to fighting.

Here, you can either shadowbox or use a bag. Personally, I prefer the second option as it allows one to give more energy into every one of his punches. Leave the fancy moves like spinning backfists and diving punches behind. Focus on straight punches and hooks. Hit the bag at full speed and power for 30 seconds. While you rest (1 minute intervals), keep your arms loose with light punches.

My Secret Weapon: MetCons

All the previous options work great and I use them quite often, but my favorite training method comes from the CrossFit world. I like to take a page out of their book and go for a **MetCon** (Metabolic Conditioning); a special type of approach that focuses, as the name implies, on your conditioning and which will turn you into a real cardio beast.

You'll be performing different exercises as fast as you can, just like regular HIIT sessions. But in this case, you'll be favoring your performance above all. The goal will be to either complete as many rounds as possible in a given time. Or a certain number of sets in as little time as you can. Which means that pacing will hold an even more important place here. There'll be no obligatory pauses, so you'll have to manage your rhythm so as to always remain in that fine line between being too slow or too fast.

I love MetCons for more reasons that I can count. For one, they're highly functional and will make you more efficient in a wide array of everyday moves. They'll keep your body guessing as, unlike other activities where you keep repeating the same routine week after week, you'll never go through the exact same workout twice! Therefore, you'll avoid that dreaded moment when the body just isn't that bothered anymore and stops improving altogether. Remember that log book where you'll be keeping a record of your food intake? Use it to track your training sessions as well (your time, your reps). You can say goodbye to those soul crushing plateaus that last for months! You'll continue to make progress for the years to come.

Another sweet benefit you'll get out of them involves the development of your muscles. MetCons contribute to their full growth by hitting those fibers in a totally different manner than strength training. The perfect complement to the latter, they'll help building a well-rounded musculature that's both powerful and dynamic.

Last but not least, as you'll notice, MetCons are a lot of fun! Once you'll have gone through a few, you'll be completely sold as to their usefulness and efficiency. You'll see that this is what challenging oneself is all about! The pleasure of pushing past your limits, the sweet taste of breaking a new PR... If Superman wasn't born on Krypton and had actually had to train to acquire his speed and agility, he'd probably have done MetCons!

Among the many exercises you can include in your MetCons, here are the most familiar and beneficial. I'll usually slap a few together, set the timer on 20, and get the party started.

Burpees: this truly is the king of all cardio exercises and that's why it deserves the first spot. Not only will burpees work your entire body, they'll send your lungs into overdrive. It's always a good idea to combine them with other movements as burpees on their own will bring you to your knees in a snap.

To perform burpees, start from the standing position. Bend down as if about to squat, and aim for the ground with your hands. Once you've laid your fingers down, throw your legs behind you to adopt a push-up position. Do one push-up. Bring your legs back close to your hands. Get up and jump.

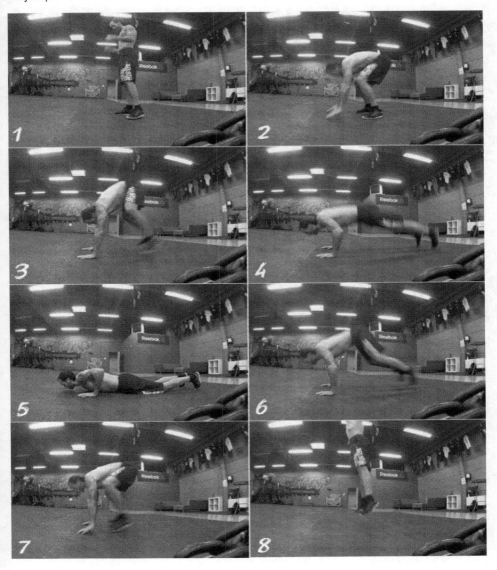

Box jumps or tuck jumps: another movement that'll test your spirit, box jumps are exactly what their name implies, i.e. jumps on a wooden box. The only subtlety lies in the fact that you need to straighten your legs at the top, after your jump. Although people typically use boxes for this exercise, you can do it on any stable object that's about 20-24 inches high. If you want, you can perform tuck jumps instead, where you jump as high as you can and bring your knees to your chest.

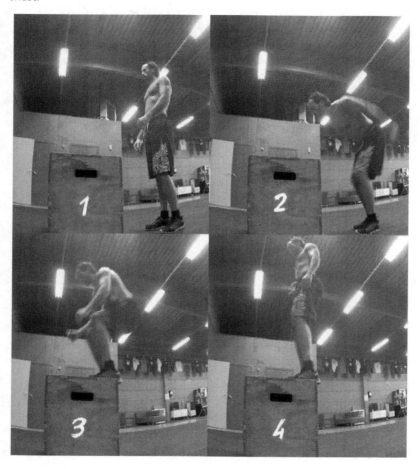

Squats: the grand-daddy of lower body exercises, squats are as basic as they come but powerful nonetheless. If they're avoided by some people, it's because they're thought to be bad for the knees and the back. However, as long as they're performed as follows, you don't risk anything. Keep your back straight throughout the exercise. Never round it. You need to understand that it's not your knees that should induce the movement but your buttocks. Your knees are merely bending as your butt goes backwards and your thighs get parallel to the ground. Think of it as you sitting down on a chair.

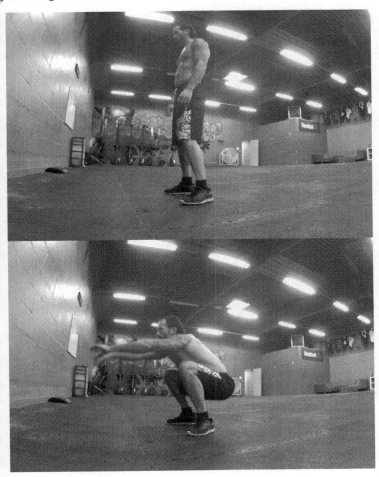

Sit-ups: no need to introduce the sit-up. Any person interested in getting in shape has tried at least a couple in his life. I like to do mine without my hands behind the head. I find that pressing your fingers on your neck can accentuate the curve of your spine to an unnatural degree.

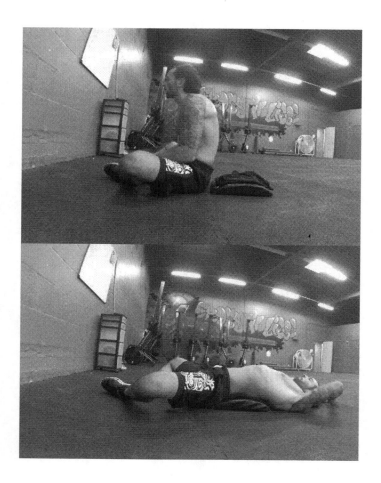

Push-ups: to count as 1 rep, your push-up should go all the way down and you should touch your chest to the ground. If you can't do regular push-ups yet, you can lean on your knees instead of the feet. Don't worry; we'll see in Part III how to increase your strength gradually to be able to perform push-ups all the way to the 1-arm variation.

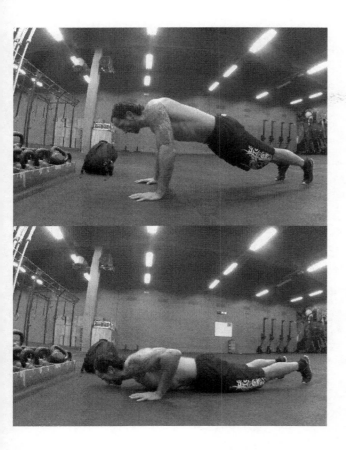

Elbow plank: one great isometric exercise, the plank will work your core like no other. Get in a push-up position and support yourself on your elbows rather than your hands. Keep the position until your abs scream for mercy.

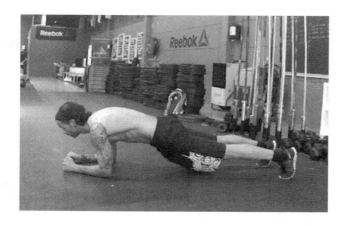

High knees: here, you'll run on the spot and bring your knees as high as you can on every step. Try to go higher than horizontal for the best results.

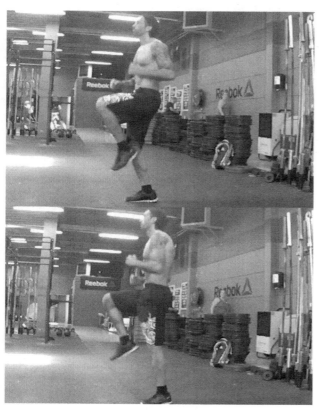

Jumping jacks: get the neon headband and tight shorts out for a trip back in time when aerobic classes were all the rage and jumping jacks reigned supreme. Standing still, you'll jump and spread your legs shoulder-width while bringing your arms to the side and having your hands meet at the top.

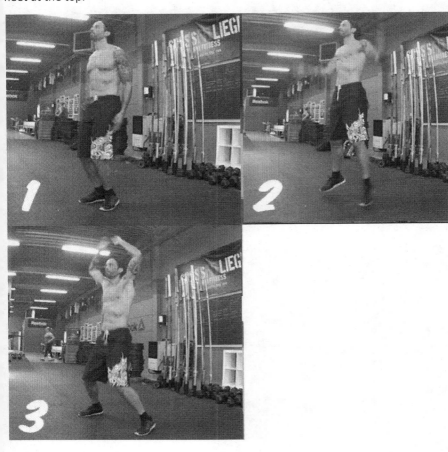

Lunges: hands on your waist with a straight back, you'll take a step forward, bend your legs, and come graze the ground with your back leg.

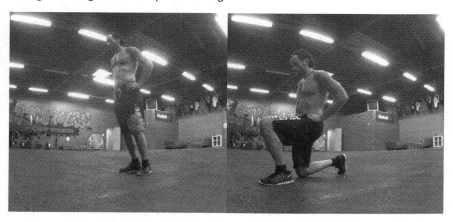

Mountain climbers: in a push-up position, bring one knee forward to the arm on the same side. Then, switch legs.

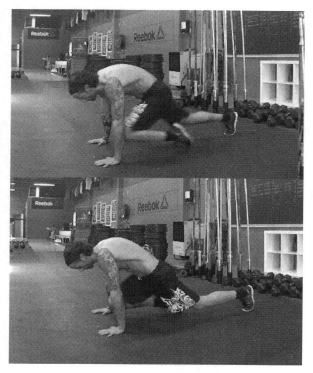

With these 10 simple movements (that you can mix with rope jumping, rowing and so on), you can create hundreds of different MetCons that'll give your body more than enough reasons to tough up and that'll get your cardiovascular system where it needs to be.

If you can't execute some of these exercises yet, as I explained before, don't fret. In Part IV where we'll lay down the actual training plan, we'll start with the basics to ensure everyone can progress all the way to the most demanding and spectacular of moves.

To give you a taste of things to come, here's a small personal selection of MetCons:

- My favorite HIIT variant goes by the sweet name of "Cindy", the infamous CrossFit WOD where you'll be trying to complete as many "5 pull-ups, 10 push-ups and 15 squats" rounds as feasible for 20 minutes. Consider yourself lucky if you still remember YOUR name once the time's up;
- Another "fun" MetCon is to row 1000m, do 20 pull-ups and 30 box jumps. Rinse and repeat 3 times;
- With burpees Tabata style, we'll go down and dirty for only a couple of minutes. But that's a short time that'll seem to drag on forever. Go burpee crazy for 20 seconds. Rest for 10 seconds. And repeat the cycle for a grand total of 4 minutes.

PART III

Build Muscle with Strength Training

"You're much stronger than you think you are. Trust me."

Superman

If I say "muscle building", what's one of the first images to come to your mind? Should it involve bunches of men packed inside a gym, staring in turns at the mirror and at the girls training on the ellipticals, you'd have a pretty accurate picture of what people usually associate with these two words.

Indeed, when looking to increase their muscle mass, most guys think their only option is to sign up for a gym membership at the nearest club... So they do, with varying results. While some do succeed in gaining a few pounds, many more fail to achieve any visible results. We've already gone over the reasons why; the lack of knowledge on their part, the improper nutrition, the absence of any real plan of attack. However, one fundamental issue is that even those who manage to beef up are not really that much better off in the end. They may look better physically and have a couple eyeballs turn their way on the beach but it's all smoke and mirrors. Chances are they've become even slower, stiffer and more easily fatigued than before. Not really the image of performance we're aiming for!

I don't know about you but I, for one, have never seen a superhero built like a tank who had the speed of an 80 years old fresh out of the hospital after a triple bypass. And I wouldn't want to be one! Realizing one's full potential isn't all about growing huge biceps and a shredded midsection. Sure, it's a nice goal to pursue but you can get there without jeopardizing your other aptitudes, so why do it?

"I'm all ears", you say. "But if gym work won't help me become faster, stronger and more jacked than 99% of the population, as you promised, what will?"

The Muscle Building Formula

In theory, it's no rocket science: to induce muscle hypertrophy, you need proper nutrition and an adequate training program. In practice, it's a bit more complicated.

If you've read this far, you know now how to eat to promote good health and achieve the first part of the mission in ensuring you provide your body with every nutrient it requires to get into an anabolic state when it matters the most. You also know, thanks to Part II, how to develop your explosiveness and agility through HIIT. So, unlike other people who start from scratch and have a gazillion pieces to put together to create a valid training plan, we benefit from a serious head start. We've already laid solid foundations for taking our body to the next level: we're working on our speed, we're eating in optimum fashion... For us, it's just a matter of picking complementary exercises that'll grow our musculature without hindering the progress we'll make on the other two fronts.

Where regular bodybuilding movements like dumbbell curls and lateral raises reduce your mobility and work too small an area to have any real impact, the exercises we'll include in our program will further develop your balance, tonicity and proprioception – on top of promoting muscle growth.

But before we jump right into those exercises, we still need to analyze, on a biological level, how muscles get bigger. Once again, the theory is obvious, but it leads to important subtleties that'll make all the difference in the end. As we described in Part I, when you load a muscle, you're actually putting a strain on its fibers which will cause the myofibrils to tear apart. It's only AFTER you've trained and your body's repair system has kicked in that the transformation may occur. The "injury" will be fixed and – as long as you've exerted the right combination of exercises, with the right weight and the right amount of rest –the fibers will become a tad thicker to prevent potential damage in the future. Great, isn't it? Yes, but only if you know how to make that process work in your advantage.

As a matter of fact, not all types of training generate the same effects, and that's the important point to take out of all this. Depending on the intensity of the exercise and the number of repetitions you manage to crank out before you reach failure, you'll appreciate dramatic differences in your results and performance.

To make things simple, we'll consider that:

- **When you work in a low rep range** (under 6 reps): you're actually training your central nervous system's efficiency through neural adaptation. Set after set, your body will learn to handle loads more easily. It's the perfect scenario for people who wish to **increase their strength**. Not so much for those who value big muscles, as hypertrophy isn't greatly promoted by low reps;
- **When you work in a medium rep range** (6-12 reps): now, the adaptation shifts from the nervous system to the cells. You'll still see some strength gains but the main beneficiaries without a doubt will be your muscles that will enlarge in response to a longer, sharp stimulation. In other words, by increasing the time under tension, you'll **force your muscles to grow**;
- **When you work in a high rep range** (+13 reps): strength increase and hypertrophy will be minimal. When you enter that territory, neither your CNS nor your muscles get enough reasons to adapt, so no alteration is needed. Such rep ranges can be of use to those searching to **augment their stamina** and endurance.

It bears mentioning that, when training our muscles, we'll always be working close to – but not completely to – failure. We'll stop 1 rep short to avoid surtaxing the nervous system and risk overtraining or injury. But if we'll leave the high reps on the side for obvious reasons, what's the best rep range to choose as far as we're concerned? We want to grow in size but we want to become stronger at the same time, so what will do?

Training with Your Bodyweight: a Versatile and Effective Tool

Not only is it possible to reconcile strength and muscle training (and get the best of both worlds), working them concomitantly will provide even better results as growing stronger will allow you to lift heavier weights which, in turn, will put even more pressure on your muscles to enlarge.

One of the most effective methods to do that will be through utilizing your own bodyweight. Compared to free weights and regular bodybuilding machines, bodyweight training offers a wide range of benefits:

- **The movements feel much more natural**: with machines, you have no say in how you perform an exercise. The trajectory is already set and the only changes you can make are slight variations in your grip or the position of your limbs. Bodyweight exercises do not impose such limitations. They adapt to your particular morphology and, with no fixed system to dictate its law, you can get a much better range of motion, a better contraction and, ultimately, greater gains (with less risk of injury);
- **There are no monthly fees or equipment costs involved**: in other words, where you have to pay to use a gym or buy a set of weights to perform bodybuilding exercises by yourself, here you don't need squat. Which makes it perfect for students or people who are on a tight budget;
- **You can do it anywhere, anytime**: one of the best pros in favor of bodyweight training is that you have absolutely zero excuses not to work out. You're not dependent on a location or the opening hours of a gym; you can do it wherever, whenever;
- **It develops functional strength**: we've already said a few words on functionality before, which is the ability to use a skill (strength in this case) in your daily life. By focusing on bodyweight movements, you'll develop the type of power that could be a life-saver in an emergency situation or that could prove useful to simplify your existence. But that's not all. You'll also increase the control you have over your body and your general sense of awareness;
- **Your joints will thank you**: bodyweight training is just superior when it comes to joint and tendon health. It doesn't put them at risk by loading them at abnormal angles with weights that may be too heavy or that may escape your grip. On the contrary, it'll make them stronger and more flexible;
- **It's a lot of fun**: this might be one subjective statement but if you've spent any amount of time in a gym, you'll probably agree that pumping iron day in, day out, isn't the most exciting thing ever. After a while, it turns into a chore, and it takes your best mental tricks to drag you there and go through the motions. It's so much more motivating to learn to master your own bodyweight. There's just no comparing the excitement of graduating to a hard progression and merely adding 5lbs to your triceps extension. Not only is bodyweight training very effective in building freakish, "farm boy" strength, it can also be very spectacular (of the kind to have people's jaw drop in awe.)

All in all, we'll choose to make bodyweight training the basis of our program because I don't want to give you any excuse to slack off, but also because that's one sort of workout that brings huge dividends and which is doable by any person with two arms and two legs. All you need to do is take the leap.

That being said, we still have no idea how this will all help us juggle with our reps range to build both strength and muscle. Can you really achieve extreme power and an impressive physique with no other weight than yours? Isn't using your body too darn easy? To answer those questions, I'll just point to professional gymnasts. Look at their herculean frame. How do you think they've built those incredible figures?

By using their own weight and applying one simple rule called: progression.

The Power of the Progression

Yes, the name of the game, as far as we're concerned, will be "progression." In short, we'll start with the easy mode of an exercise and we'll progress through more and more complex variations as our body becomes stronger. We'll do that by reducing what we call our mechanical advantage. One of the techniques we'll use will be to position ourselves in such a way as to bring our gravity center further and further away from where we're applying the force. We'll thus need more strength to produce the same result.

As an example, it's much easier to perform a push-up on the knees as it is with the whole body straight; simply because – through extending your body – you've increased the tension at the support points (that is the shoulders).

The beauty of progressions is that they're never totally identical from one to the next. With bodybuilding exercises, the motions stay the same; you simply slap on another plate when it gets too easy. Here, the angles and body stance may vary from step to step, which means that your muscles and central nervous system will be stimulated in entirely different manners, which is great for gains. Every time you improve, you keep challenging the muscles by hitting them from another angle. Improvements in balance and coordination will also arise.

How to Progress

Building our reps up to 12 before switching to a higher progression will be the key to this program. Usually, if you want to speed through the progressions as fast as possible, you can make the shift once you've become strong enough to perform 6 clean reps. But in so doing, you're always putting maximum tension on your joints; you're draining your system by performing at extreme intensity without ever giving it a break.

This may be OK at first but, eventually, if you keep pushing that hard, something bad is bound to happen. By waiting until you're able to pass the +10 reps mark, not only will you give your body the opportunity to adapt, you'll mostly give it time to train within the best rep range for muscle growth!

In other words, we'll be **increasing our strength** as we tackle the new progression for a couple of weeks and barely manage to get a few reps in, **and our muscle mass** as we get better and able to stay at it for more reps.

That's the way to go for optimum gains on all fronts! That's the way we'll be heading down.

The Exercises

Like most people, when I first began training towards muscle hypertrophy, I didn't see the whole picture. I was only interested in developing my "beach muscles"; those that make you look good when strolling down that golden patch of sand along the sea...

In other words, I was neglecting my lower body, and it showed! I didn't know it at the time but – more than creating an off-balance, weird-looking chicken legs physique – shunning the legs trongly impeded my progress. I was limiting my evolution by not training the biggest muscle roups, responsible for the biggest testosterone spike!

)nce I added leg drills to the mix, I saw a huge difference in my overall development. Even my pper body widened.

o get a well-rounded, superhero-like physique, you can't omit to work any single body part. 'ou might be tempted, as I was, to focus on chest development and the obtainment of big guns, ut not only would it prove to be a waste of your time, should you succeed in getting the upper)ody of a Thor, you'd look ridiculous with your sticks for legs. You need to be the complete)ackage to realize your true potential. From head to toes.

ach muscle group will be trained either directly – if we're dealing with a large one – or ndirectly in case it's too small to really matter. Remember what we said about dumbbell curls ind the likes? One of the reasons they're not the best bang for your buck is because they work oo specific an area. For biceps and triceps, it's better to favor movements that will involve)ther, larger muscles at the same time. Muscles like the pecs or the lats.

)ne last precision before we delve into the heart of the matter; where we focused on intensity 'or cardio, here we'll ensure we get enough rest between our sets to make every one of our -eps count. Does it bear mentioning that, prior to your first session, you should test your skills to ;ee at what progression to start? I didn't think so.

Without further ado, here are the exercises we'll be tackling in our program, along with their many variations:

Push-Up Progressions

I know what you're thinking: I must be joking, right? As if push-ups could hold the key to a superman body! If that's what you believe, I'll admit that you're indeed correct... up to a certain point. We often hold that idea because we can't see past their regular form. And if you stick to those, you may grow a little, but it's true that you'll never become part of the 99th percentile.

Once you've outgrown that progression and it has stopped providing enough resistance, it's simply a matter of reaching for a more advanced step as described below. Push-ups in all their tinges and colors will be perfect to develop your pushing power as well as rock solid pecs and triceps.

Incline Push-Up: the first progression in this series, incline push-ups can be practiced on any elevated surface which offers stable hand support. If the wall can do for a start, you'll want to move to items closer and closer to the ground, until you're near the horizontal.

As for the push-up in itself, with your back straight, lower your torso all the way down, then push with your hands to return to your initial position.

Knee Push-Up: no more wall or bench to ease the process here, but your muscles will still get a break thanks to your knees that'll help limit the tension at the shoulder level.

Just perform the push-ups while supporting your weight on your hands and kneecaps.

Regular Push-Up: now, you're going to engage your entire body. From the starting position – body straight and hands shoulder-width apart –, come down until your chest hits the ground. Then come back up.

Hand Release Push-Up: you'll increase the difficulty by releasing your hold once you touch the floor. In other words, once your torso makes contact, lift your hands off a few inches, put them back on the ground and push yourself up.

Diamond Push-Up: decrease the leverage by placing your hands one next to the other (thumb against thumb) and changing the angle of your arms with respect to the floor. This progression will put a greater stress on the triceps.

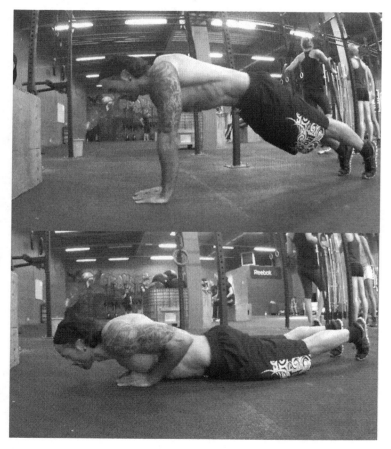

Decline Push-Up: want even more pressure on your pushing muscles? Get your feet elevated. The higher your legs, the harder it'll be.

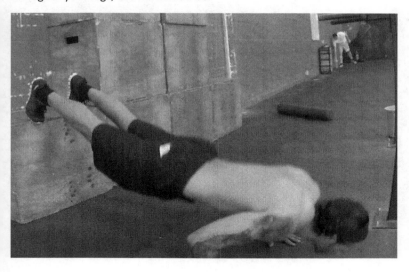

1-Arm Incline Push-Up: same as the incline push-ups described above... but with 1 arm.

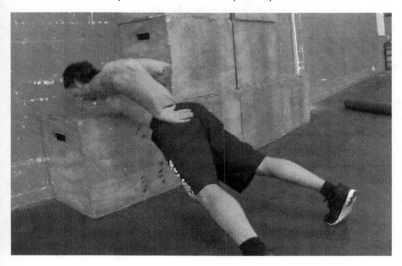

Archer Push-Up: this progression will prepare you for the 1-arm push-up by increasing the weight you have to support on a single hand. To do an archer push-up, spread your hands wide. But instead of bringing your body straight down like usual, go to the right or the left and come place your ribs against the hand on the corresponding side.

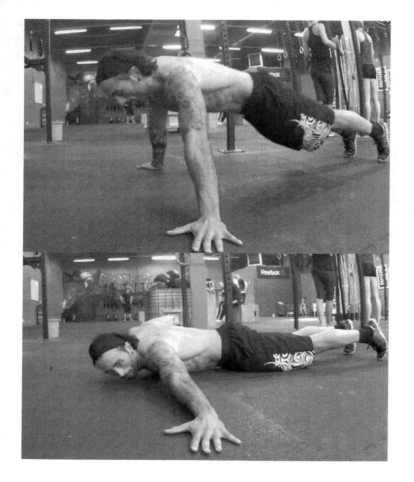

Here, you'll want to get your hands further and further apart until there's only one that does most of the pushing and the other is only there for support and to help stabilize your body.

1-Arm Push-Up: the name says it all; perform the push-ups with only 1 hand on the floor. You should pay attention to your position during this exercise. Make sure that you keep your back straight, your elbows to your flanks, and that your chest doesn't turn to the side when you lower your body.

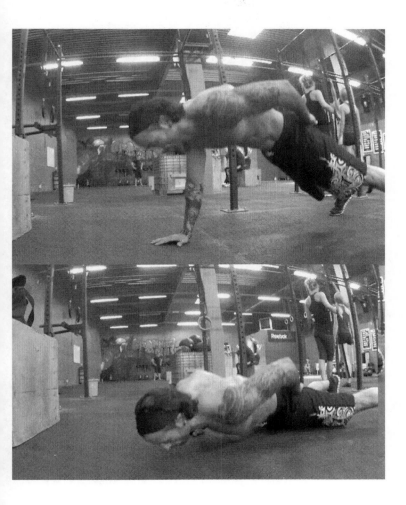

For a start, you can keep the legs spread apart for better balance but, eventually, you'll need to get them closer to perform the progression perfectly.

Once you've mastered this step, you can still increase the difficulty by removing the number of fingers in support, 4, 3, 2, 1…

Pull-Up Progressions

The pull-up is to the back and the biceps what the push-up is to the pecs and the triceps: that is the best exercise to target those muscles. Once again, we'll start with easy progressions that'll soon get harder and harder until we reach the holy grail of pulling exercises: the 1-arm pull-up.

Every exercise below can be performed either in supination or pronation (that is with your palms facing you or facing away.) The first option is the easier one and will therefore be avoided as it won't result in the best gains possible.

As for where to do your pull-ups, I'd say anywhere you can hang from: a tree branch, a swing, a soccer goal... If you have 20 bucks to spare, you can also buy a bar that'll fit inside your door frame. That'll be the best $20 you've ever spent.

Eccentric Pull-Up: if you can't yet do a standard pull-up, don't worry. You can make your body gradually stronger by working on the eccentric part of the movement. Use a chair or any other such object to get your head over the bar and grab it. Then, let your legs hang and try to control the descent.

Jumping Pull-Up: here, you'll start the pull-up with a slight jump that'll give you enough momentum to get your head over the bar.

Half Pull-Up: your body hanging from the bar, pull yourself half way and go back to the starting position. As it gets easier, go higher and higher until you manage to put your chin over the bar.

Regular Pull-Up: self-explanatory. Make sure you go all the way down before you attempt another rep. Don't be like those guys who think they're real beasts, pumping thirds of reps.

Wide-Grip Pull-Up: with a wider grip, you'll increase the torque on your back muscles. Fully warm-up the shoulders before attempting this variation as it'll put a lot of tension on your joints.

Chest-to-Bar Pull-Up: to execute a C2B pull-up, you need to continue pulling and not stop until your sternum has touched the bar.

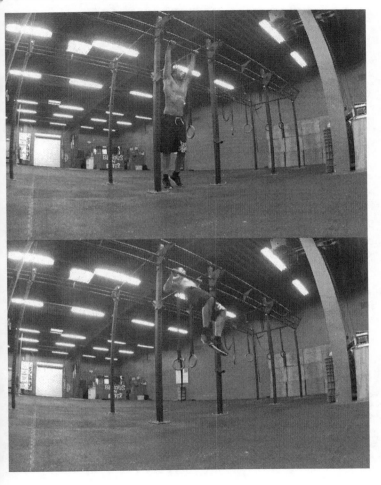

Archer Pull-Up: Same idea as for the archer push-up but applied to pull-ups. You'll grab the bar with a wide grip and pull yourself up to one side.

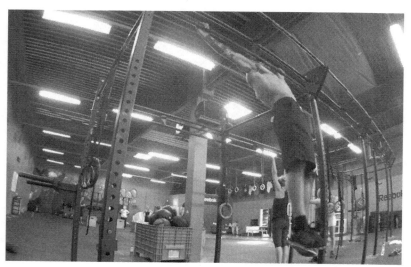

1-Arm Eccentric/Jumping Pull-Up: once you've become strong enough, you can choose either eccentric or jumping pull-ups with one arm to further strengthen the joints and get you ready for the last progression.

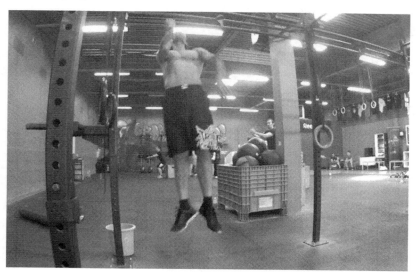

1-Arm Pull-Up: relatively speaking, the 1-arm pull-up is much harder to accomplish than the 1-arm push-up but that shouldn't deter you from pursuing that amazing skill (personally, I'm still working on it.) As with the 1-arm push-up, you'll want to keep your arms close (read glued) to your side to gather as much strength from the lats and the biceps as possible.

Squat Progressions

I already introduced you to the wonderful world of the squat in Part II where I described the basic progression that almost everyone who starts out should be able to do.

Once you can churn out a good dozen without fail, it's time to turn to more advanced variations that'll help turn those skinny legs into real oak trees.

Bulgarian Split Squat: elevate one of your feet (on a bench, a bed, a piece of furniture) to put more stress on the front leg that will perform the squat. The move will feel somewhat like a lunge but significantly harder.

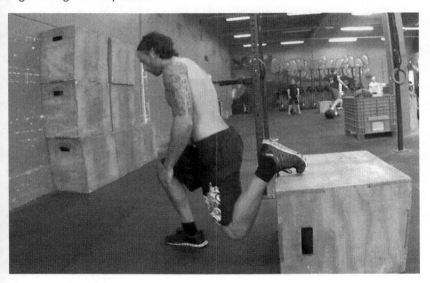

Side-to-Side Squat: spread your legs wide apart (about twice your shoulder width) and get down on one side as you would on the hands for an archer push-up.

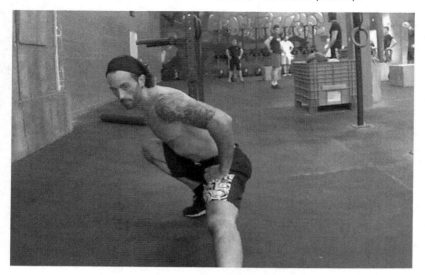

Box Squat: this time, it's the working leg that'll find itself raised in comparison to the support leg. Standing on top of a box or any other such item, place your rear foot on the front side of the object and let it slide down as your front leg contracts into a squat position.

Pick an item which height allows you to use your rear foot at the bottom to build some momentum for your front leg.

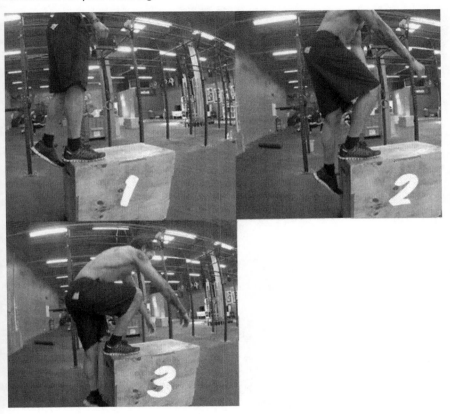

Assisted 1-leg Squat: grab on to a chair or a post while keeping one leg straight a few inches off the ground in front of you. Now, lower yourself as much as possible with the other leg. Go deeper and deeper until you've gone through your whole range of motion.

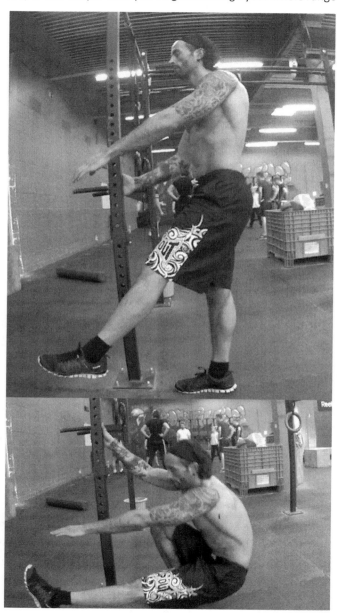

High-heel pistol Squat: prior to trying your legs at the pistol squat, get entirely ready with this easier variation of the move. Stick something under your heel, like a book or a wood block of about 2 inches, before going all the way down on that leg. That'll help in relieving some of the tension.

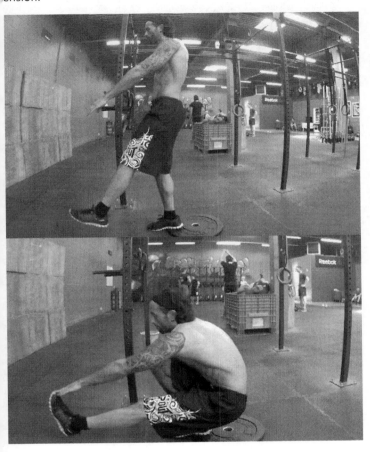

Pistol Squat: you've got nowhere to run and no bar to hold on to anymore; just get on one foot and do your thing! Balance is often an issue when starting out. To make it easier on yourself, extend both arms in front of you. And watch that back!

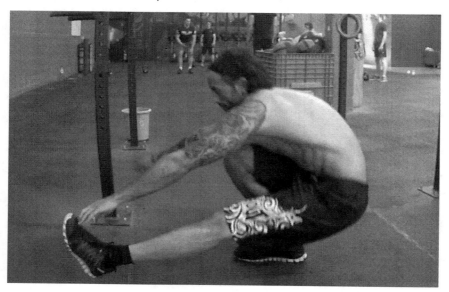

Handstand Push-Up Progressions

You've always admired broad shoulders that inspire respect? You want to develop yours and get that nice rounded shape? Then, this series of exercises is for you.

Handstand push-ups will make you stronger, more balanced and flexible at the same time. But first, if you are to get to that point, you need to learn to stand with your head upside down. The best way to start is with a headstand; that's where you use your head on the ground as extra support. Just kneel down next to a wall, arrange the top of your head and your hands so that they draw a triangle on the floor, kick your legs up and – with your feet resting on the wall – try to keep your balance in the air.

Once this move becomes comfortable, it's time to begin the real work.

Handstand Hold: same move as the headstand but you'll take the head out of the equation. Now, your entire weight will rest on your hands, and you will feel it. By building your holds to a few dozen seconds, you'll increase your power and reinforce your wrists and tendons.

As much as possible, when drilling handstands, try to keep your body straight. In a perfect world, it should make a straight line from your head to your feet.

Pike Push-Up: with pike push-ups, you'll get a feel of things to come. Get in a push-up position but with your feet closer to your hands (keep the legs straight) in such a manner as to make an inversed V-shape relatively to the floor. As you bring the feet closer and closer, you should feel more tension on your shoulders. That's good. Now, without flaring the elbows too much, perform the pushing motion.

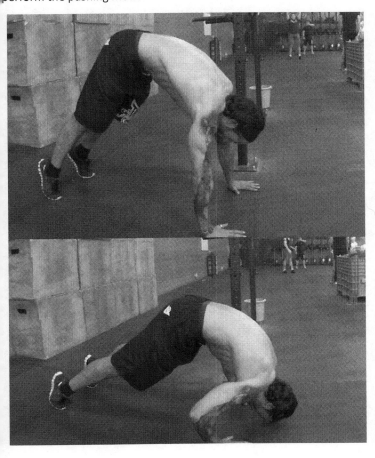

Elevated Pike Push-Up: to increase the weight on your hands, elevate your feet as you would for a decline push-up. The difference here is that you'll keep the break at the hips to ensure it's the shoulders that get most of the load and not the pecs.

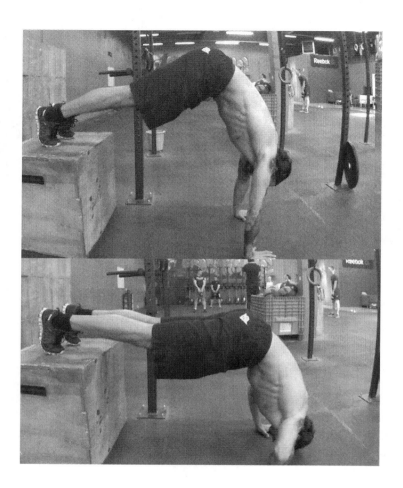

Kipping Handstand Push-up: an easier variation of the handstand push-up, the kipping HSPU will use the momentum from your hips to help raise that body up. You can consider it's the equivalent of a jumping progression for exercises where your feet are on the ground.

In a headstand position (thus with head and hands on the floor), with your lower back resting on the wall, bend the knees in front of you as if doing a squat... Then, explode with your hips, throwing your feet up and pushing with your hands at the same time. Bingo.

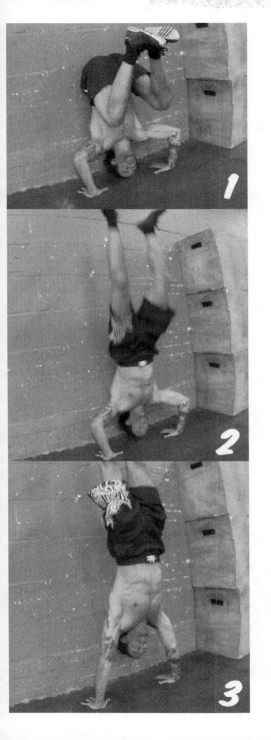

63

Standard Handstand Push-Up: you've worked this far for this; so you know what to expect. Get in a handstand against the wall and, with your body in a perfect line, go down with your shoulders and press back up when you've reached the bottom. Here, more than ever, your form is critical. Arching the back will prove detrimental to your progress as it'll allow other muscles to jump in and help, thus making the exercise less efficient.

Deep Handstand Push-Up: for a bigger challenge, increase your range of motion by elevating your hands. By resting the latter on a raised surface like books or parallettes, you will allow your head to go deeper than the horizontal. Which will result in more tension, which will mean more strength and muscle gains. You can limit yourself to the eccentric part of the progression at first to get used to the greater ROM.

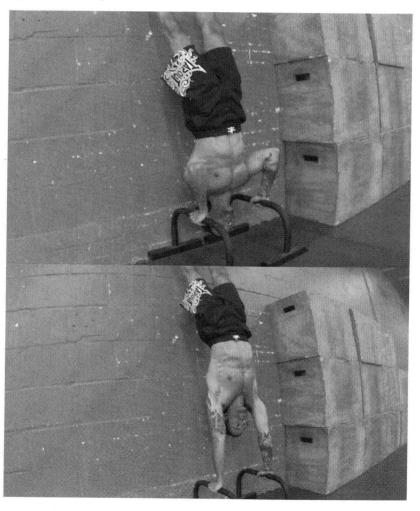

Rowing Progressions

We already have a great strength and muscle builder for the back and the guns in the pull-up. But all the progressions leading to the 1-arm pull-up target the lats and biceps in the same way. That is, the force is always applied in a vertical plane, never horizontally.

That's why it's great to supplement those exercises with the following progressions that'll fill the gap and ensure you not only develop those muscles fully but also strengthen your core.

Vertical Pull: grab a post or the handles of a door and, with your feet next to that object, lean back so that you feel the stretch spread throughout your back. Now, pull yourself towards your hands until your chest makes contact.

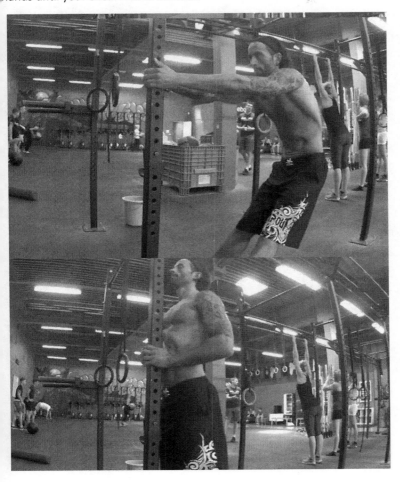

Inverted Row: the pulling technique remains identical but, with your spine facing the floor, you'll put even more stress on your lats. To begin with, start with the legs bent. And straighten them as it gets easier.

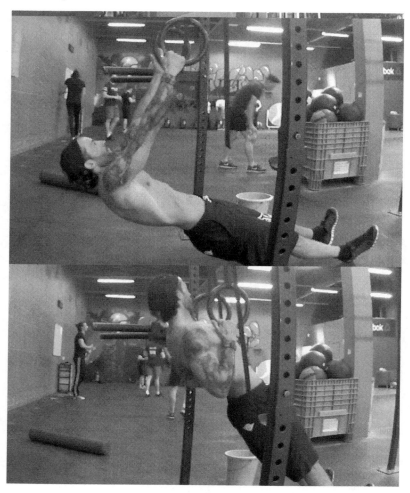

Tuck Front Lever Hold/Pull-Up: the front lever progressions that follow will be hard not only because, when you get your body in such positions, you seriously decrease your back's mechanical advantage, but also because you might be limited by your core strength if it happens to lack even slightly. However, you can expect that, if you stick with them, they'll build tremendous power in those areas.

The first progression towards the full front lever is the tuck front which requires that you get the hips and shoulders on the same plane, horizontal to the floor, with your feet up in the air. For this variation, tuck your knees to your torso and round the back. You want to be as tight a ball as possible to limit the tension on the lats.

When you can hold the movement for a solid 10 seconds, you can execute pull-ups in that position to further engage your muscles.

Advanced Tuck Front Lever Hold/Pull-Up: now and until the last progression, we'll be aiming to extend those legs further and further away from our chest, which will greatly increase the difficulty as our weight shifts further and further away from under our arms.

For the advanced tuck, we'll simply "unround" the back. You'll notice that such a small change can have dramatic effects on your ability to perform. If you experience any trouble with this position or the former, try to pull down with your shoulder blades when grabbing the bar and pulling your legs up. This will help in activating the right muscle chain.

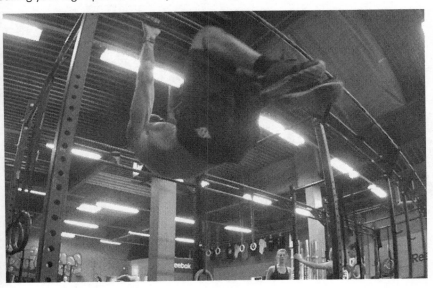

Straddle Front Lever Hold/Pull-Up: so far, you've progressed by moving those knees away from your center 1 inch at a time. When you feel ready, get your legs straight in front of you and spread wide apart.

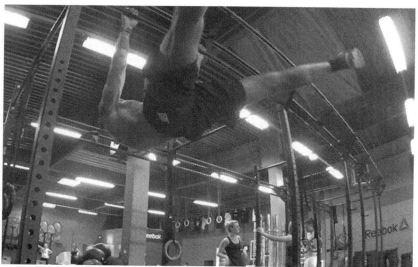

Front Lever Hold/Pull-Up: to go from straddle to full front, it's not a matter of moving the knees away from the torso anymore but rather of closing the legs. Little by little, reduce the spread until your legs are one next to the other and your body is totally straight from shoulders to toes.

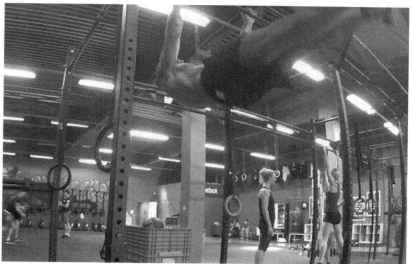

Don't forget to add pull-ups to every one of your progressions for a complete stimulation.

L-Sit Progressions

If your idea of sculpting abs of steel involves hundreds of sit-ups and crunches, you're about to have your worldview shattered. Sure, sit-ups can be useful in a MetCon or to build your core's endurance. But to develop real power, you'll have to resort to an isometric/static hold that goes by the name of L-Sit.

More than creating an impressive midsection, L-Sits will build your compression power, your rear shoulders strength, as well as wrist control and flexibility. It'll also be useful to reach the type of strength needed for your front lever.

Tuck L-Sit: though every progression here can be performed on an elevated surface, I recommend you stick to the floor as it's the more difficult version. For the tuck L-Sit, take position with your hands on the ground, facing sideways, and your arms straight.

Push down to raise your butt off the floor, and use your abs to bring your knees close to your chest. Remain in that position for as long as you can.

1-Leg L-Sit: here, you'll keep one knee up and extend the other leg in front of you.

Standard L-Sit: your body is now in the shape of an L (hence, the L-Sit name) with both legs straight and parallel to the floor.

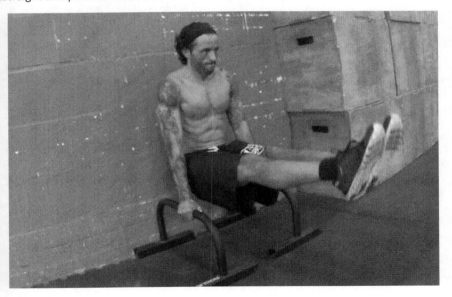

V-Sit: to decrease your leverage and thus increase the difficulty, you'll be lifting the legs gradually so that the angle between them and the floor rises all the way to 90°. As your legs get higher, you'll feel it more in the triceps.

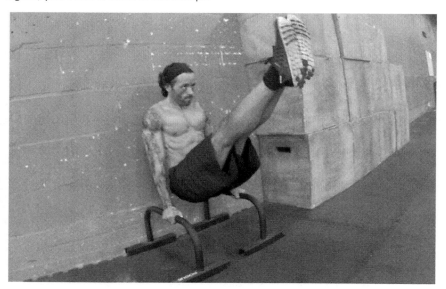

Handwalk Progressions

This exercise, when it gets to the later progressions, can be performed by either moving yourself forward with your hands (that's why it's called "handwalk") or with any rolling device like an ab wheel or a loaded barbell. It'll serve as a nice complement to L-Sits for forging the ideal six-pack.

Plank: a beginner move, the plank can be useful to prepare your abs if you've never exercised before or if you're still lacking core strength. To achieve a plank, just get in a push-up stance and hold it until your abs give in. Piece of cake.

Elbow Plank: by lowering yourself on your elbows, you'll be putting more stress on the core. Try and hold it for at least 20 seconds at a time.

Knees Handwalk: when you feel ready for this progression, adopt the same position as for a knee push-up. Instead of diving straight down though, you'll be bringing your head and chest to the floor by walking your hands forward one after the other. Once fully extended, simply walk back to the starting position. As always, watch that back!

Incline Handwalk: for this one, you'll start from a regular push-up position. However, going from a knee to a full handwalk is too wide a gap to cover at once. That's why you'll include an intermediate step in training your handwalk at an angle.

Find a sloping street or a wooden plank that you can use to create a level difference in favor of your hands, and walk on that. You can also, if that progression proves to be too much of a challenge, complete partial reps until you manage to extend completely.

Full Handwalk: no more knees or slope; with your body straight, walk forward until your forehead touches the floor, then come back and do it again.

This concludes a list of progressions that should sure keep you busy for a while and make your entire body grow like a wild plant in the Amazonian forest. If you apply every technique described here above and show the necessary tenacity, you WILL get fit, muscular and powerful.

With that being said, if your aim stretches beyond mere fat loss and the development of a beach-worthy physique – if you won't accept anything short of the very best version of yourself you can be –, you'll need to supplement your program with some barbell work.

The Little Extra that Makes All the Difference

Like I said, bodyweight exercises represent the bulk of our training. They will – on their own – make you better than 99% of the people around you... I'm not going back on my word, rest assured. So if you don't have access to a gym, it's definitely OK; you can still develop superhuman strength and a great body.

But for those who want to reach their full genetic potential, I still wanted to include a small chapter that revealed the 3 best barbell exercises to add to your weekly program to really push the envelope.

I've chosen these particular exercises for several reasons. For one, they engage large muscle groups which will allow us to lift heavy (and secrete a lot of testosterone.) Then, they complement our current regimen perfectly by targeting more of the lower body – which may get in a rut once you've mastered the pistol squat.

Unlike bodyweight progressions where the mechanics differ from variation to variation, with these 3 there's only one technique to learn for each. Once you've nailed them, it's just a matter of putting more and more weight on the bar.

Back and Front Squat: normally, you shouldn't have too many problems here as you've worked the movement over and over again in your HIIT or bodyweight sessions (refer back to the squat section above for a refresh on the proper form to use.)

For bar placement, you have the choice between using a front rack position – that is, while holding the bar by your fingertips, to lift your elbows up in such a manner as to have the barbell rest across your shoulders along your collarbone. Or the usual back squat position where the barbell lays on your trapezius. I leave the option up to you but, even though I prefer the front squat as it's more technical and demanding, the back squat is the alternative that can support the heaviest loads. Thus, go for the back squat for the biggest gains.

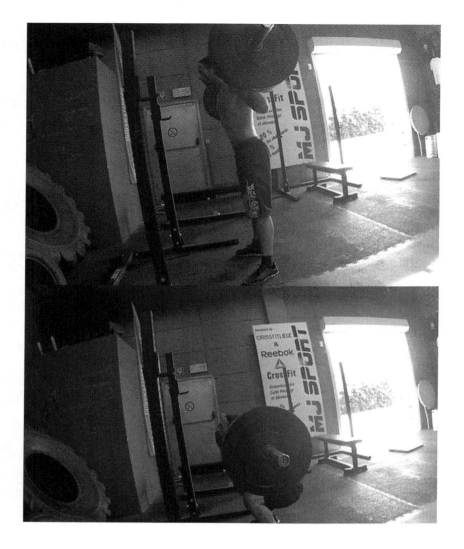

Deadlift: in short, to perform a deadlift, you'll pick the barbell off the floor, push with your legs and straighten your back. As with the clean & press, though it looks easy, it's much more technical than it appears to be.

Start with your feet slightly spread apart and your shins against the barbell. Grab the load with a shoulder-width grip and bend down as if doing a squat. The key to a successful deadlift is to initiate the movement with the legs and buttocks. Push with your heels until the barbell has reached past your kneecaps before you pull with your lower back.

Never allow it to arch! You might injure yourself seriously. Here, more than ever, start light. Drill the movement until it becomes second nature before you go up in weight.

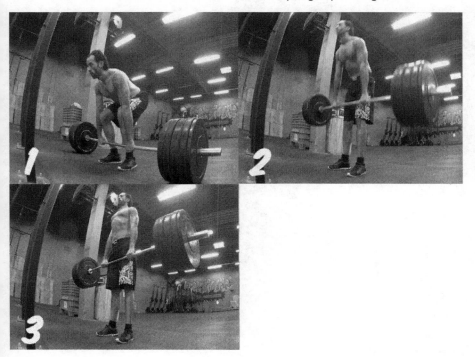

Clean and Press: the clean & press deserves a spot on this list because, like the deadlift, it works more than half a dozen different muscles. It also brings tremendous power and speed.

This highly dynamic exercise combines two fundamental movements – the clean and the press, duh! That's where it gets a little tricky as the transition between the two needs to be very smooth... which isn't the easiest thing when you're just getting started.

To perform this exercise, start as you would a deadlift; that is grab the bar and push on your legs to get it off the ground. And once it gets past the knees, explode with your hips while doing a shrug to have the barbell shoot upwards. Slightly bend the knees as you get under the bar and adopt the rack position similar to a front squat.

Now, with the bar resting on your shoulders, it's press time as you push that load overhead. Once you've cleared the head, make sure you realign your spine to maintain your balance and fully engage your shoulders.

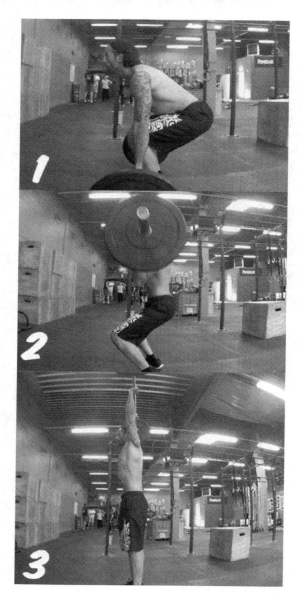

Congratulations, you've now seen everything you need to know to become faster, stronger and more jacked than anybody else around you. All we have left to do is to assemble that knowledge into a cohesive program. In other words, to lay down a plan of action for you to follow and grow from. Alright, you're ready? Let's turn you into a real life superman!

PART IV

Putting It All Together –
The 100 Days Plan to a Super You!

*"It's time to begin a new cycle. A new life.
One that I can control. One that I can live with.
It's time to let go of the past. It's time to
create something new. Something of my own."*

Wolverine

This is it, the part you've been waiting for! We now have all the pieces of the puzzle to get on our way and build ourselves a solid program. I'll take you by the hand and show you, for the next 100 days, what to do (and why) in order to reach your goal of building the perfect body.

Why 100 days? Because that's how long it takes to see concrete results that'll last but also because forming new habits doesn't happen overnight. You'll have figured by now, this is no "lose 20lbs and get a six-pack while you sleep" type of program that promises the moon and the stars but ends up delivering crap. It'll take time and efforts on your part, but it'll be hours and sweat very well spent; I can guarantee you that!

We want you to create a new routine that you'll ease into and slowly integrate as an inherent part of your superhero life, like sleeping, taking a shower or kicking ass. After that period, if you've successfully hung on, you won't even have to make a conscious effort anymore; you'll just eat how you're supposed to and train without having to argue with yourself about it.

Obviously, your program won't suddenly stop once those 100 days are behind you; you'll want to continue reaping those life changing benefits. But you'll have made enough progress by then to be able to manage on your own without my help. You'll have built a lifelong habit that'll take you to the top!

The First 2 Weeks

What You Can Expect
The first 15 days are very particular in that your motivation will probably be at an all-time high, which should give you a much needed hand in sticking to this program. But at the same time, those days will be amongst the hardest you've known because of your nutrition. On one side, you'll have just finished reading this book and you'll be all pumped up, ready to take on the challenge... On the other, you'll find yourself in detox literally as your body adapts to its new source of energy (fat) and comes off the sugar.

This will create an unstable balance where anything can happen. You won't feel good at first and you need to get prepared for that because, if you're not, you might give up at the slightest discomfort, thinking that this is how you'll feel all along. So, I want you to understand that it does get better afterwards. No, let me take that back; not only will it get better, you'll soon feel fresher and more alive than you've ever felt! But before that, you need to feel lousy. There's no way around it.

You'll feel weak, irritable and light-headed. You may even experience withdrawal symptoms like headaches and nausea, depending on your level of dependency. Strong cravings for sugary foods will also come and torment you as your body rids itself of this poison. But even those urges, however sharp they may be, will eventually subside. In short, you need to tough it up and push through. The pot of gold lies at the other side.

The Walking Dead
For all these reasons, we'll start slowly as far as physical training goes and we'll get you through these first 2 weeks with as little distress as possible. You'll be in no shape to undergo any

ntensive program head on, so no strenuous efforts for you. At this stage, putting even more stress on your body and your mind would only serve to break you. As your organism switches to fat-burning, you'll be taking walks, and that's the only exercising you'll be doing. "What?" you say. I know, you didn't buy this book to get told to stroll around like a zombie and take it easy; you want some action! To which I would answer: don't be so hasty, my little friend. After a few days of following your new diet, you'll be thanking me you're not doing MetCons yet! Besides, it may not look like much (after all, even the most out of shape people, the very antithesis of superheroes can do it without as much as breaking a sweat) but walking brings a lot to the table.

For one, being easy doesn't mean "no efficiency". Calories WILL be burned, and in a calm and stress-free manner to top it off. You can thus go at it for long periods and not suffer the same detrimental effects as with prolonged cardio. Walking will also be gentle on your joints (unlike running), especially if you still have some weight to shed. And your knees and ankles will get a chance to strengthen before you graduate to more intense forms of training, as will your leg muscles. Though you'll never build massive thighs and calves hiking through the woods or walking your dog, it can help to invigorate underused muscle tissue and get it accustomed to a little more than the usual trip from the couch to the fridge.

And the pros keep piling up... The simple fact of putting one foot in front of the other for any length of time will positively affect not only your blood glucose but also your triglyceride levels. What about your immunity system? Heck, it'll give it a boost too!

Walking will also teach you a thing or two about the paleo precept of living in the present. While you're going through your miles, take in the scenery, breathe deeply, try and notice the small beauties of this world. In a lot of ways, this practice resembles meditation; it can be a time to stop, think and reflect. Which can prove invaluable if you're the creative type in need of some inspiration.

The first week, you'll be taking 3 walks of 30 minutes each. If you want, make arrangements to work that time in your current schedule by, for example, walking to the office/school instead of driving there. Or dedicate extra time on the side to do it. Do as you please, as long as you can stick to it.

For week 2, depending on how you feel, increase that time up to an hour at once. Remember: don't kill yourself just yet. The main purpose of these 15 days is not to get you fitter per se; it's to have you run on a much better fuel! Speaking of which, what will we be eating during those 100 days?

Your Groceries List

In a way, dressing a list of foods to eat isn't so much about determining what to include as it is what to keep out. As we discussed at length, grains, legumes and sugar packed foods will definitely get a no-go. So, in essence, as long as you avoid those, anything is permitted.

I know, leaving you at that wouldn't help much. When I started out, I had a good hold of the theory but, still, I had no idea where to begin or what to do. That's where a small, typical groceries list can come in handy. To give you some guidelines on what to buy to keep your belly happy, here's what I usually get from one week to the other.

Don't hesitate to subtract from or add to it depending on your particular tastes, as long as it stays true to our "rules." Also, don't forget to use the tips I shared with you in Part I to try and lower that bill as much as possible.

Meat

- Ground beef;
- Beef tenderloin;
- Pork chops;
- Fish (salmon, cod, basa, halibut);
- Prawns;
- Chicken drumsticks;
- Chicken breast;
- Canned tuna in olive oil;
- Cans of wild salmon;
- Bacon.

Vegetables

- Zucchinis;
- Eggplants;
- Broccolis;
- Artichokes;
- Brussels sprouts;
- Tomatoes;
- Peppers;
- Celery;
- Carrots;
- Asparagus;
- Mushrooms;
- Olives (black and green);
- Onions;
- Garlic;
- Packaged salads;
- Frozen veggies.

Fruits

- Avocado;
- Lemons;
- Kiwis;
- Bananas.

- Nuts (almonds, pistachios, brazil nuts, pecans);
- +80% dark chocolate;
- Dried fruits;
- Dates.

For both fruits and snacks, you'll want to watch your intake and use them with moderation, especially at the beginning of your journey. Unlike meat and vegetables which you can eat to your heart's content, nuts are highly caloric and not as filling. Handfuls have soon disappeared down your throat and you've just absorbed a thousand calories!

As for fruits, though they contain vitamins and are good for your health, they also hold sugars that will cause your insulin to spike.

Dairy & Eggs

- Grass-fed butter;
- Free-range eggs;
- Goat cheese.

All that food would taste quite bland without the following, which I keep in my cupboard and use to cook and prepare my yummy meals: extra virgin olive oil, coconut oil, black pepper, salt, cayenne, cinnamon, garlic powder, paprika, turmeric, coriander, chives, basil, ras-el-hanout...

Sample Recipes

Now that you have your basic blocks, all you've left to do is to pick a few and to mix them any way you see fit. You don't need to become a master chef to eat right. Most of these ingredients work perfectly well together, which gives you hundreds of possible combinations. And, most importantly, they're easy to cook.

To give you a leg up and generate some ideas, here are a couple of my own "achievements" even a child could make.

Pork chops with broccoli, bacon and garlic

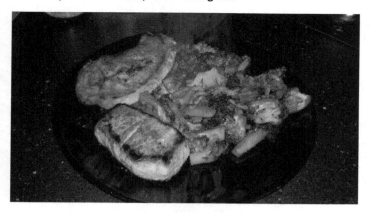

Salmon fillets with zucchini and eggplant

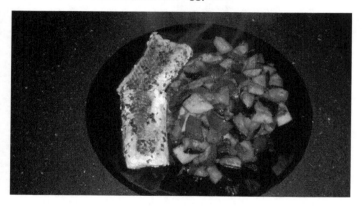

Lamb chop with mushrooms, leeks and artichokes

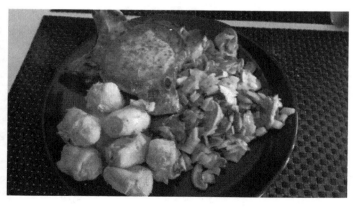

Beef stew with red and green bell pepper, celery, eggplant, curry and coconut milk

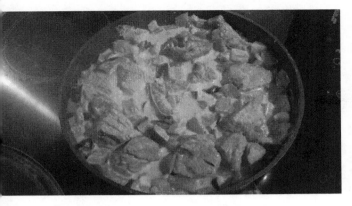

Chicken breast with carrots, broccolis, cauliflower and zucchini

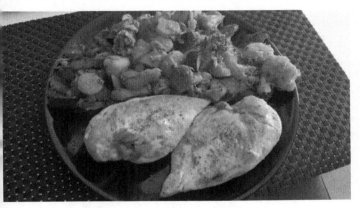

Omelet with 5 whole eggs, chives and chicken strips

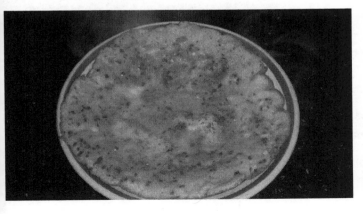

Monster salad

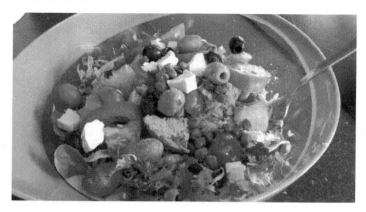

Banana pancakes (1 egg mixed with 1 mashed banana)

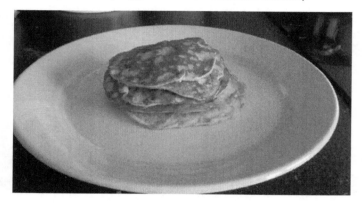

You don't really need detailed instructions to make any of these meals. For most, just heat the pan sufficiently, pour the oil/fat of your choice to grease its surface, add the veggies you've chopped beforehand, season with salt and spices. Let it all cook until brown (usually about 15-20 minutes) while stirring every now and then, and preparing your meat on the side. Bon appétit!

The only recipe that requires a little more explaining is the beef stew, and still it's a piece of cake to make. First, start cooking the chopped peppers and celery, wait until they've softened up before adding the eggplant. During that time, brown the pieces of beef in another pan. Once seared, transfer the beef to the veggies pan and add the curry and the coconut milk. Bring the milk to a boil, then reduce heat and simmer for 20-30 minutes.

With our way of eating, there's no more clear distinction between breakfast, lunch and dinner. Where the majority of people eat cereals, bread or pancakes in the morning, a sandwich at noon and a hot meal at 6/7p.m., sometimes you'll find yourself eating the leftovers of yesterday's frittata or having smoked salmon and an avocado for breakfast – to give you an example.

You'll become more flexible. Not by exerting a hard and conscious effort but simply because that's how paleo transforms you. Before I made the switch, I would never have imagined a breakfast without a big bowl of sweet, crunchy cereals. For me, the two went hand in hand; cereals WERE what made a breakfast! Today, not only am I off the sugar and its evil grip, my taste buds have never been so delighted with all those healthy fats and natural products I'm exposing them to. Every meal is now an occasion for celebration.

Week 03 - Week 07

If you've held on so far, let me congratulate you on a job well done. Though we still have a long road ahead of us, the hard part is now behind you. By the third week, most of the fatigue should have gone away. Your body should have made a partial switch to fat burning and you should feel energized and ready to take the world by storm. I don't need to spare you anymore.

As soon as you feel your strength coming back, you'll add HIIT sessions to your program. As before, we want to go gradually to prepare your body properly and build strong enough foundations to move forward in the best and most secure manner.

Week 03 to week 07 will serve to make you fitter and lighter, increase your body awareness, and teach you how to properly do squats and other such exercises that we'll build upon later on.

How many times will we be training? We'll **keep with our 3 weekly workouts**. Although I strongly suggest you don't stop taking your long walks, HIIT will be what we focus on for the next month.

Refer back to Part II for the full list of exercises. As much as possible, you'll want to work every part of your body at least once a week and always include squats as well as push-ups in one form or another.

Here are the sessions I propose to start with for your first 4 weeks of HIIT.

High Knees

This easy workout is perfect for making the transition to high intensity training. For 10 rounds, you'll be following this pattern:

30 seconds high knees – 15 seconds rest;

30 seconds high knees – 30 seconds rest.

Once it stops being a challenge, increase the number of rounds or decrease the resting period.

Whole Body Workout

Here, you'll be alternating 3 exercises for a total of 8 rounds, without any rest:

16 basic squats;

8 push-ups;

16 mountain climbers.

Burpees Hell

10 seconds burpees – 10 seconds rest;

20 seconds burpees – 20 seconds rest;

20 seconds burpees – 20 seconds rest;

30 seconds burpees – 30 seconds rest;

40 seconds burpees – 50 seconds rest;

40 seconds burpees – 50 seconds rest;

30 seconds burpees – 30 seconds rest;

20 seconds burpees – 20 seconds rest;

20 seconds burpees – 20 seconds rest;

10 seconds burpees – 10 seconds rest;

10 seconds burpees – over.

Another variation to try out (when you'll have developed good enough bases) is to alternate 20 burpees with running 200 yards. And to do it 5 times, as fast as possible and without any rest in between.

Hill Runs

Find an uphill slope of a few degrees and:

Run to the top (time yourself);

Walk back down to catch your breath;

Wait 2x your run time;

Repeat for 10 minutes.

Jumping Workout

For 6 short rounds, do this as fast as you can:

15 jumping jacks;

20 high knees;

10 box jumps.

Half-Cindy

As described in Part II but for 10 minutes "only", do as many rounds as possible of:

5 pull-ups:

10 push-ups;

15 squats.

Mix-It Up

Try to complete 7 rounds of the following while going hard:

10 burpees;

15 sit-ups;

20 lunges.

Isometric Workout

Here, we'll be performing static exercises to work our muscles differently.

Get in a handstand position against a wall for 15 seconds;

Drop in a squat and remain at the bottom position for 10 seconds;

Elbow plank for 20 seconds;

Hang from a pull-up bar for 15 seconds;

Do it 8 times.

Short but Brutal

For 6 minutes, do the following:

10 tuck jumps;

5 hand release push-ups (or any other PU progression you can manage);

20 sit-ups.

Death by Squat

20 seconds squats – 20 seconds rest;

30 seconds squats – 20 seconds rest;

40 seconds squats – 20 seconds rest;

Repeat the pattern 5 times.

Week 08 - Week 11

From week 08, you can introduce tubers into your diet (sweet potatoes, yams and the likes). The quantity and frequency will obviously depend on your fat levels and your goals. A nice recipe for sweet potatoes is to cut them in long sticks, lay them on a tray, sprinkle some salt and paprika, add a dash of olive oil, and bake in the oven for about 30 minutes (425°F). And there you have yummy fries that'll bring a wide grin to your face!

The big step we'll take during this period will be the **introduction of strength training**. I know, at last! You'll also need to beware because that's where the motivation from the start usually starts to wane. So you have to keep focused and remind yourself why you're doing all this (for some tips on how to stay motivated, I'll see you back in Part V.)

How will we be implementing those exercises in our current schedule? We'll simply add them to our 3 weekly HIIT/MetCon sessions, right after the warm-up. The reasoning behind this is that: on one hand, we want to be as fresh as possible to work on our strength and build muscle; so they must come first (whereas cardio training remains highly valuable, even if we don't perform at our "bestest.") On the other, we don't want to do them on separate days or you would find yourself with 6 days of training per week, which wouldn't be quite as manageable.

Bodyweight Training Routine

If you don't have access to an Olympic barbell, this is how you'll be organizing your training:

1st day: work on your progressions for the push-up, the squat and the L-Sit (+ HIIT);

2nd day: work on your progressions for the handstand PU, the pull-up and the L-Sit (+ HIIT);

3rd day: work on your progressions for the squat, rowing and the handwalk (+ HIIT).

You'll be doing 5 sets of each. As for the number of reps, as you probably remember, build it to +10 before you move on to the next progressions.

Bodyweight Training Routine, with Barbell

If you do have access to an Olympic bar, this is how to adapt your schedule accordingly:

1st day: work on your progressions for the push-up, the pull-up, the squat and the L-Sit (+ HIIT);

2nd day: work on your progressions for the handstand PU, rowing and the handwalk (+ HIIT);

3rd day: work on your heavy lifts (+ HIIT).

For the heavy lifts, you'll apply the same method; that is 5 sets of 6-12 reps. And an increase in weight once you get over those numbers. As a reminder, the exercises you'll be working on are: the barbell squat, the deadlift and the clean & press.

Week 12 - Week 15

As far as nutrition is concerned, there won't be any radical change for week 12. The only difference will be the possibility of intermittent fasting. After 3 months of using this program, your body's chemistry will have changed in ways you would have never believed, and including this last tool to your plan will further help complete your transformation.

Just to be clear: fasting is on a voluntary basis. It'll provide other great benefits to your following the paleo principles... but you can still achieve your goals of a great physique without it. If you choose to pursue that path, I'd recommend a 24 hours fast, once a week. In other words, skip breakfast and lunch, and only have dinner. Nothing overly complicated.

For the training part, if that's doable, I would add a fourth session (personally, I think 4 workouts a week is the best frequency; it allows the fastest improvements while also leaving enough rest for you to recover and come back stronger.)

With 4 sessions, you can now activate the cruise control and enjoy the ride that will lead you all the way to the perfect body. For a 4 days program, I advise the following split:

1st day: handstand push-up, barbell squat (+HIIT);

2nd day: push-ups, deadlift (+HIIT);

3rd day: pull-up, clean & press, l-sit (+HIIT);

4th day: rowing, handwalk, squat.

And if you don't use a barbell, make it so that you train every progression twice per week.

Phew, we did it! That was a lot of information for you to digest but you pushed through and you made it. Attaboy! You know everything you need to turn your regular self into a real life superman. Now, it's "only" a matter of implementing this method and really giving it a chance, of using the momentum you've built to get you going and growing. You can choose to do nothing and wait for a better time to start (which will never come). Or you can take action today and realize your every dream.

The ball is in your court.

PART V

Fine Tuning –
Settling the Last Details

"No matter where you turn,
there's a decision to be made.
Life or death. Right or wrong.
Regular or crunchy."

The Punisher

f after reading the last chapter, you still have questions that remain unanswered, I invite you to oin me in this ultimate part where I discuss the few points yet hanging.

Q&A

Question: Is age a big factor when trying to get in shape?

Answer: Are you too young or too old to build muscle mass and become a model of athleticism? I'm not going to lie; if you're under 15 or over 50, you'll have somewhat of a harder time reaching those goals than a guy in his prime. But it shouldn't deter you from trying. You see, though it's generally believed that our metabolism takes a dive as we get older, it actually decreases by less than 1% every ten years! It's no excuse not to work out. In fact, it's because we don't take care of ourselves and don't train that we become soft and slow in our later years, not the other way around!

As for being too young to follow this program; there's a tenacious myth which states that working your muscles at an early age will stunt your growth. It's just not true! In fact, it may even improve it as your growth hormone production gets stimulated by the training.

Question: Should I train on an empty stomach?

Answer: This is one of those topics that show ardent supporters in both camps. Some argue that doing any type of physical activity without eating first is bad because your body will go straight for your muscles and cannibalize them. Others insist that it's the greatest thing ever because, with you being in a fasted state, your glycogen levels will have dropped quite low, allowing you to burn fat more easily.

In our case, it doesn't really matter who's right or wrong. As we don't rely on carbs as our primary source of energy anymore, we're already drawing from our fats – whether training or not! Which means we don't really need to run or work out on an empty stomach. Should we choose to do it though, contrary to people who still enjoy their grains, our muscle tissue will be preserved. And to make matters even better, we'll be able to train as if our tank was full; that is at full power without any loss in performance.

Question: How many hours of sleep should I be getting?

Answer: You've probably heard of successful men and women who manage to get by with only 4 to 5 hours of sleep a night, and you wonder if you couldn't maybe follow in their footsteps. Imagine all the time you'd have on your hands to pursue your passions and enjoy life if you didn't have to spend so much of it lying down in total unconsciousness! Unfortunately, I'm sorry to bring you the bad news, but that's one area where you absolutely can't compromise!

When you sleep less than 7-8 hours per day, you're starting to put stress on your organism. You might not feel it at first but that stress will build up, and up, and slowly tear you down if you do nothing about it. Your progress will stall; you won't gain any muscle... Worse, you might even see your body fat rise as your hormones get thrown out of balance!

Rest is a critical part of leading a healthy and prosperous life. As the saying goes, you don't grow when you work out but rather when you're sleeping, as that's when the body gets a chance to rebuild the damage you've done. So make sure that you catch enough Z's if you're serious about realizing your goals.

Question: Do I need supplements to progress?

Answer: Browse through any bodybuilding magazine and you'll see hundreds of supplements touted as the world's greatest discovery guaranteed to take you from zero to hero. You have protein powders, gainers, creatine, BCAAs, glutamine, prohormones... supplements that end up costing an arm and a leg to people who try to keep up. Thank God, we won't need any of those.

Through our meat-heavy diet, we're already getting all the protein we require to build quality muscle. We don't even have a use for a multi-vitamin with all the veggies and fresh fruit we're eating daily. In short, we've got everything covered to be in perfect health and thrive; so don't waste your money buying supplements that pale in comparison to the nutrients already available through your food. If you want to make an investment, purchase grass-fed beef or organic vegetables. Good food is all you really need.

Question: How to ensure I don't overtrain and how to tell if I am?

Answer: If you're following this program to a T, you shouldn't have anything to worry about as far as overtraining is concerned. Working out 3 to 4 times a week should give your joints and muscles plenty of time to recover in between sessions. However, if you're neglecting your sleep or your diet, you might begin to feel some of the following symptoms: a soreness that doesn't go away, bad mood swings, frequent sickness, a total loss of motivation, insomnia, decreased sex drive...

If you encounter any of those signs, kill the problem dead in its track before it does any long term damage. Cut the training for a week or two (only leave the walks) and ensure that you sleep and eat enough. If you want to take preventive measures, you can choose to plan a deload period every 8 weeks to give your system time to regenerate. During that week, don't do any strenuous effort; drop the weight on your lifts, go back a few progressions for your bodyweight exercises, reduce the number of sets, and take it easy on the HIIT and MetCons.

This also means that you should stick to our 3-4 days split. Don't train more, thinking that it'll get you faster to your destination. I know all too well – as the extreme person that I am – that when you want something bad, you might be tempted to overdo it. But you'll just end up getting side-tracked.

Question: What about training when I'm sick?

Answer: I used to think that it was OK to train when I didn't feel very well. No matter how sick I was, I didn't want to miss any workout and risk stalling my evolution, so I went anyway and trained. I didn't know that I was, in fact, hurting my progress! It took longer for my body to heal; my performance became subpar, and I spent a lot more time in sickness having to deal with this weakened version of myself! In other words, don't do it. Get well and resume training only when recovered.

Question: How to deal with injuries?

Answer: If, despite all your precautions, you still get injured, don't make the mistake of rushing back to training too soon. I'm a firm believer in the RICE formula as a way to deal with any soft tissue damage. When you get hurt, **R**est the affected area, **I**ce it, use **C**ompression and **E**levate it. All those measures are meant to reduce the inflammation and get you back in the saddle ASAP. If it looks anything near serious, consult with your GP. Don't mess with your health.

Question: What's the best method to warm-up prior to training?

Answer: A proper warm-up is the best way to remain injury-free. It'll prepare your body for the efforts to come. As such, it should be gentle and progressive, and it should produce a light sweat.

To get ready for my training sessions, I usually like to skip rope at a slow pace, run a few hundred yards and/or mix a couple of light exercises like jumping jacks and high knees. After that, I prep my joints with swings and rotations. All the joints get their fair share, from the neck to the ankles. Stretches are best left for the end of the workout, just before heading to the shower.

Question: How can I stay motivated throughout this program and beyond?

Answer: First, you need to understand that there's no one-size-fits-all answer to this question. In fact, there are as many possible replies as there are people interested in undergoing this type of training.

You're bound to have moments where you feel down and could think of a thousand things you'd rather be doing than lacing up your shoes and going for a HIIT session. It'll happen; it always does. And that's why you need to find what I call your "prime drive". That's what will keep you hanging on when the going gets tough. If you sit back, close your eyes and start reflecting on the reasons that pushed you to read this book, what can you come up with?

You need to dig deep. Don't just accept the first thought to come to mind like "to look better when I go to the beach, this summer." If you think about it long enough, you'll end up finding your real drive; the one that's hiding behind all the false motives you've built to protect yourself. Because oftentimes we're hurting, and we tell ourselves and others lies as the truth is too hard to bear.

Maybe you've always felt insecure because of your extra weight, and you'd like to develop your body to find a sense of confidence. Maybe you've always felt like you were meant for greatness but you never achieved anything because you never really gave yourself the adequate tools. Maybe you want to get stronger in order to protect your loved ones, or get more stamina to enjoy your kids for the decades to come – and not die from a heart attack 10 years from now because you'll have abused your body a little too much. Or maybe you're just fed up with feeling like crap and not having enough condition to walk a single flight of stairs. Whatever that reason, once you've found it, put it down on paper. Flesh it out. Describe what it is you're trying to accomplish and how it'll change your life once you do.

Better yet, accompany that paper with a collage of inspiring pictures that you'll hang in evidence in your room as a constant reminder of your goals and aspirations. Use images of people or heroes you admire, of items you wish you would own, of places you'll visit once you've made it. Now is not the time to be meek or to censor anything. Don't put any limits in front of you.

Dream BIG so you can become larger than life!

Conclusion and a Little Bonus

There you have it, my 100 days program to make a superhero out of you! By the end of these 3 months, if you ate and trained as we've seen, you should find yourself faster, stronger and more muscular than ever before. And with a lust for life you never even conceived!

After a while, you'll notice your abs starting to pop out. As your body stabilizes around the 10% body fat mark, you'll develop a constant 6-pack that'll show whether you're "flexing" or not. You'll look great and perform like a champ. This level of fat is not only very pleasing to the eye, it's also optimum for health and efficiency. That's where we're aiming to settle.

But maybe that's not enough for you. When you searched for your prime drive, maybe you found that what you wanted was a ripped physique that went even beyond abs and power. If that's your case, if your desire is to get even more shredded than superman himself, check out this special report I made for you. In it, I share my secrets to go lower than 10% and reveal every fiber of muscle that lies beneath your skin.

To download your free report now, visit: http://reallifesuperman.com/freereport/

Let's Keep in Touch

Now that this book comes to an end, I'd like to extend a hand to you. I feel like we're somehow connected now. I hope that the content of this guide resonated with you and your past experiences, that you could identify with my journey, my ambitions and setbacks. If that's the case, no matter where you are in life today, we're kindred spirits with yet a lot to share!

That's why I'd like to keep in touch; so we can continue to progress together. We've both embarked on a road that knows no end, a road to perfection that can sometimes get very lonely when no one else around you can relate. We can offer each other that support. We can help each other become better!

Whether you have a question to ask, a comment or suggestion you'd like to make, or if you simply want to tell me about your goals and the progress you've already made, you can reach me via my site:

Real-Life Superman: http://reallifesuperman.com

It'll be my pleasure to help! Speaking of help, if you have 2 minutes to spare, I'd like to ask for yours. I need your feedback to find out if I'm on the right track. I've tried to lay down everything I know about training and getting in the best shape of your life but it's still a work in progress. I know it can still be improved. That's why I'd like to hear what you have to say about it. If you could do me a favor and drop a word or two about this book on Amazon, it would mean the world to me!

I thank you in advance and I'll see you soon, my friend.

About the Author

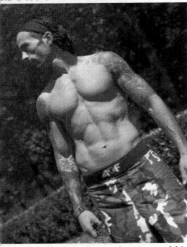

A black belt in Karate, ring-tested kickboxer who also holds a university degree in Psychology, I have to admit I know a thing or two about kicking butt and imposing my will on my foes. However, the real adversary I've always been looking to vanquish – whether in CrossFit competitions, in a race or a fight – has never been anyone else but me.

I believe in the Latin phrase *mens sana in corpore sano* and try to honor that spirit every chance I get by looking for new, more efficient ways to improve myself and reach the next level. Through my trials and errors, I've accumulated a vast wealth of knowledge. Not only on the **quickest means to attain one's physical peak** but also on what it takes to toughen up mentally and develop a sharp, indestructible mind.

In this series of books, I intend to share with you everything I've learned in close to 20 years of studying and perfecting my training. It is the next natural step for me: to put into words all that baggage made of sensations, hard-earned habits and unspoken truths; to extract its very essence without holding anything back. And by so doing, not only will I get better, you will as well!

Some of the facts I'll lay out will surprise you, others may come as a shock, but rest assured that they represent the **fastest shortcut to success**. So, if you're ready for the change of a lifetime, let's get started and discover the Superhero who had been hiding inside you all along!

Sincerely,

Markus

Made in the USA
San Bernardino, CA
07 August 2015